YOGA

YOGA

Emmanuel Carrère

Translated from the French by John Lambert

FARRAR, STRAUS AND GIROUX

New York

Farrar, Straus and Giroux
120 Broadway, New York 10271

Printed in the United States of America
Originally published in French in 2020 by P.O.L, France
English translation published in the United States by
Farrar, Straus and Giroux
First American edition, 2022

Library of Congress Cataloging-in-Publication Data
Names: Carrère, Emmanuel, 1957– author. | Lambert, John, 1960–
    translator.
Title: Yoga / Emmanuel Carrère ; translated from the French by John
    Lambert.
Other titles: Yoga. English
Description: First American edition. | New York : Farrar, Straus and
    Giroux, 2022.
Identifiers: LCCN 2022014035 | ISBN 9780374604943 (hardcover)
Subjects: LCSH: Carrère, Emmanuel, 1957– —Mental health. | Authors,
    French—20th century—Biography. | Authors, French—21st century—
    Biography. | Yoga—Therapeutic use. | Manic-depressive illness. |
    LCGFT: Autobiographies.
Classification: LCC PQ2663.A7678 Z46 2022 | DDC 843/.914 [B]—
    dc23/eng/20220426
LC record available at https://lccn.loc.gov/2022014035

Our books may be purchased in bulk for promotional, educational, or
business use. Please contact your local bookseller or the Macmillan
Corporate and Premium Sales Department at 1-800-221-7945, extension
5442, or by email at MacmillanSpecialMarkets@macmillan.com.

www.fsgbooks.com
www.twitter.com/fsgbooks • www.facebook.com/fsgbooks

10 9 8 7 6 5 4 3 2 1

If you bring forth what is within you, what you bring forth
will save you. If you do not bring forth what is within you,
what you do not bring forth will destroy you.

—Apocryphal Gospel of Thomas

Contents

I

THE ENCLOSURE

The arrival

Seeing as I have to start somewhere in relating the story of these four years—during which I tried to write an upbeat, subtle little book on yoga, was confronted with things as downbeat and unsubtle as jihadist terrorism and the refugee crisis, was plunged so deep in melancholic depression that I was committed to the Sainte-Anne Psychiatric Hospital for four months, and, finally, during which I bade farewell to my editor of thirty-five years, who for the first time wouldn't be there to read my next book—I choose to start with this morning in January 2015, when, as I finished packing, I wondered whether I should take my phone, which in any event I wouldn't be able to keep with me where I was going, or leave it at home. I selected the more extreme option, and no sooner had I left our building than I was thrilled to be under the radar. It was just a short walk to the Gare de Bercy, where I'd catch my train. From this annex of the Gare de Lyon, small in size and already quite provincial, dilapidated train cars take you straight to the French heartland. The old-fashioned compartments, with six first-class and eight second-class brown and gray-green seats, reminded me of the trains of my distant childhood in the sixties. A few army recruits slept stretched out on the seats, as if no one had told them that military service had been abolished long ago. With her face turned toward the dusty window, the only person near me watched the graffitied buildings file past under a fine gray rain as we left Paris and passed through the suburbs to the east. She was young, and looked a bit like a hiker with her huge backpack. I wondered if she was on her way to go trekking in the Morvan hills, as I'd done long ago, in weather conditions that weren't any better than they were today, or if she was going—who knows?—to the same place I was. I'd made up my mind not to take a book, and spent the trip—an hour and a half—letting my eyes and thoughts wander in a sort of calm impatience. Without knowing exactly what, I was expecting a lot from these ten days I'd spend cut off from everything, out of contact, beyond reach. I observed myself waiting, I observed my calm impatience. It was interesting. When the train stopped at Migennes, the young woman with the big backpack also got off, and, along with me and twenty or so other people, headed over to the square in front of the station where a shuttle bus would pick us up. We waited in silence, seeing as no one knew anyone else. Everyone sized up everyone else, wondering if they looked normal or not. I would have said they did, or at least normal enough. When the coach pulled up, some sat down together, I sat alone. Just before we left, a woman in her fifties with a handsome, solemn, sculpted face climbed in and sat down beside me. We said quick hellos, then she closed her eyes, indicating that it was fine with her if we didn't talk. No one spoke. The coach soon left the town and headed down narrow roads, crossing villages where nothing seemed open—not even the shutters. After half an hour it turned onto a dirt road lined with oak trees, and stopped on a gravel driveway in front of a low farmhouse. We got off, picked up our bags from the luggage bay, and entered the building through separate doors, one for the men and one for the women. We men found ourselves in a large, neon-lit room fitted out like a school dining hall, with pale yellow walls and small posters bearing bits of calligraphed Buddhist wisdom. There were some new faces, people who hadn't been in the coach and who must have arrived by car. Behind a Formica table, a young man with an open, friendly face—dressed in a T-shirt while everyone else was wearing either sweaters or fleece jackets—welcomed the new arrivals one by one. Before going up to him we had to fill out a questionnaire.

The questionnaire

After pouring myself a glass of tea from a big copper samovar, I sat down in front of the questionnaire. Four pages, back and front. The first didn't need much thought: personal information; people to contact in case of emergency; medical situation, medication, if any. I wrote down that I was in good health but that I'd suffered several bouts of depression. After that, we were invited to describe: (1) how we'd become acquainted with Vipassana; (2) what experience we'd had with meditation; (3) our current stage in life; (4) what we expected from the session. There was no more than a third of a page for each answer, and I thought that to seriously tackle even the second question I'd have to write an entire book, and that in fact I'd come here to write it—but I wasn't about to mention this. Prudently, I stuck to saying that I'd been practicing meditation for twenty years, that for a long time I'd combined it with tai chi (putting, in parentheses, "small circulation," so they'd know I wasn't a complete beginner), and that today I combined it with yoga. However, I didn't practice regularly, I went on, and it was to get a better grounding that I'd enrolled in an intensive session. As to my "stage in life," the truth is that I was in a good way, an extremely favorable period that had lasted almost ten years. It was surprising, even, after so many years when I would unfailingly have answered this question by saying that I was doing very, very badly, and that that particular moment in my life was particularly catastrophic, to be able to answer candidly, even playing down my good fortune, that I was doing just fine, that I hadn't suffered from depression for some time, that I had neither love nor family nor professional nor material problems, and that my only real problem—and it certainly is one, albeit a privileged person's problem—was my unwieldy, despotic ego, whose control I was hoping to limit, and that that's just what meditation was for.

The others

Around me are fifty or so men, in whose company I will sit
and be silent for ten days. I eye them discreetly, wondering
who among them is going through a crisis. Who, like me,
has a family. Who's single, who's been dumped, who's poor
or unhappy. Who's emotionally fragile, who's solid. Who
risks being overwhelmed by the vertigo of silence. All ages
are represented, from twenty to seventy, I'd say. As to what
they might do for a living, it's also varied. There are some
readily identifiable types: the outdoorsy, vegetarian high
school teacher, adept of the Eastern mystics; the young guy
with dreadlocks and a Peruvian beanie; the physiothera-
pist or osteopath who's into the martial arts; and others
who could be anything from violinists to railway ticketing
employees, impossible to tell. All in all, it's the sort of mix
you'd find at a dojo, say, or in any of the hostels along the
Way of Saint James. Since the Noble Silence, as it's called,
hasn't yet been imposed, we're still allowed to talk. As night
begins to fall, very early and very black behind the misty
windowpanes, I listen to the conversations of the small
groups that have formed. Everything revolves around what
awaits us in the morning. One question comes up again
and again: "Is this your first time?" I'd say about half the
group are new, and half are veterans. The former are curious, excited, apprehensive, while the latter benefit from
the prestige that comes with experience. One little guy
reminds me of someone, but I can't say who. Since I'm a
negative sort of person, my attention focuses on him. With

a pointed goatee and a wine-toned jacquard sweater, he's annoyingly smug in the role of the smiling, benign sage, rich in insights into chakra alignment and the benefits of letting go.

Teleportation in Tiruvannamalai

The first time I heard about Vipassana was in India, in the spring of 2011. To finish my Russian adventure novel *Limonov* I'd rented a house in the former French enclave of Puducherry, where I stayed for two months almost without talking to a soul. I started my days, which invariably followed the same routine, reading *The Times of India* in the only café, as far as I knew, where you could get an espresso. Then, following the streets that intersect at right angles and which, lined with run-down colonial buildings, bear names like Avenue Aristide Briand, Rue Pierre Loti, or Boulevard Maréchal Foch, I walked pensively back to the house to work on my book. I went to bed very early, around the time when the innumerable stray dogs in Puducherry would strike up a chorus of barking in which I could make out a few voices, and I got up very early too, woken by the first rays of dawn and the croaking of geckos. This sort of homey routine, without visits to museums or monuments or touristic obligations, is my ideal trip abroad. One time, however, I did go to Tiruvannamalai, which is a hot spot of Indian spirituality because that's where the grand mystic Ramana Maharshi lived and taught, and where his ashram is still located. The hot spot made a very bad impression on me: a fairground of gurus and spiritual seminars that attracts hordes of gaunt, grimy, fake Western sadhus oozing both pretension and suffering. Now when people who practice yoga talk to me about retreats in India where they hope to benefit from the ancestral teachings of the great masters, that's what I think of. For me Tiruvannamalai and Rishikesh—said to be the cradle of yoga—are the places where you stand the least chance of benefiting from the teachings of a great master: as little chance, say, as you do of meeting an original artist on Place du Tertre at the top of Montmartre in Paris. Bertrand and Sandra, the only two friends I'd made in Puducherry, had given me the address of a French guy who lived there. Dressed in a lilac-colored robe, he was called Didier but he had people call him Bismillah. When I asked him about his spiritual journey, Bismillah told me that one big step for him had been a Vipassana training session: ten days of intense meditation that, as he said, really cleaned out your head. As I practiced meditation in my own small way and on the face of it wasn't against getting my head cleaned out, I was curious. However, I was a little put off when I found out that on the next step of his spiritual journey Bismillah had come to Tiruvannamalai attracted by a seminar on teleportation. He'd been disappointed, he said. That left me thinking. Teleportation consists in traveling instantaneously from one place to another, simply through the power of your mind. Disappearing, say, in Chennai, and reappearing the next moment in Mumbai. A variant of that is bilocation: being in two places *at the same time*. Several traditions credit such exploits to a few rare, distinguished saints,

such as Joseph of Cupertino. But religious authorities—to
say nothing of scientists—remain cautious on the subject.
I couldn't help wondering if a guy who registers for a public
seminar on the Internet in the hope of having such an
experience—a bit like signing up for a day of scuba diving
in the hope of seeing manta rays—demonstrated exemplary
open-mindedness, or whether to swallow such a load of fiction, and then to say you're disappointed, you had to be a
bit of an idiot.

My room

The question of accommodation worries me. There are individual rooms and shared rooms, and of course I'd prefer
a room by myself but I imagine so would everyone else,
and I have no reason to say I need one more than anyone else. In another setting money would solve things: the
best rooms would go to those with the most money and I'd
have nothing to worry about. But here we're put up free of
charge. The teaching, the room and board, it's all free. All
they do is suggest you make a donation at the end, as much
as you're comfortable with and without anyone knowing
how much you've given. There must be another criterion.
The order of arrival? Or they draw lots? Or it's completely
random? When I'm done filling out my questionnaire and
take it over to the nice guy who's collecting them, I ask
him about it with an amused, complicit little smile, in the
unlikely case that it depends simply on his goodwill. No,
he tells me, also smiling, they don't draw lots: the rooms

are assigned according to age. The single rooms go to the most elderly participants. So I don't have to worry after all. The nice young man gives me a key, which I take, and I go out into the soaked garden behind the main building. To the left there's the big empty hall where we'll spend ten or so hours a day for ten days, to the right three rows of pre-fab bungalows. Mine's in the first row. Just over a hundred square feet, linoleum floor, a single bed—under it a plastic box with sheets, a blanket, and a pillow—a shower, a sink and a toilet, a little closet: the strict minimum, all perfectly clean. And well heated, which is important in the win-ter in the Morvan region. The only source of light, apart from the window in the door with a pull-down blind, is a frosted glass globe on the ceiling. It's not what you'd call cozy, I'd have liked a bedside lamp, but seeing as we're not supposed to read . . . I make my bed, put my things in the closet: warm, comfy clothes, thick sweaters, jogging pants, slippers, this is no time for vanity. My yoga mat. A little terra-cotta statue representing the Gemini twins. Five inches tall, with full, round curves: a woman I loved gave me this discreet fetish, which I take with me wherever I go. No books, telephones, tablets, or any of their chargers. When we spoke, the nice young man asked if I had any such objects to leave in storage: lockers are provided. I an-swered proudly that I'd left all of that at home. Is everyone as compunctious in following the instructions I'd received when I signed up two months earlier? Fine, we'd signed and agreed to do without such distractions and not com-municate with the outside world for ten days. But if we cheat, who'll find out? It would surprise me if they made spot checks and confiscated any books or phones people had snuck in.

Or perhaps they would?

North Korea?

Vipassana sessions are the commando training of meditation. Ten days, ten hours a day, in silence, cut off from everything: hard-core. On the forums, a lot of people say they're satisfied with, and sometimes even that they were transformed by, such a demanding experience. Others denounce them as a sort of sectarian indoctrination. The place is like a concentration camp, they say, and the daily meeting a form of brainwashing, with no room for discussion, to say nothing of disagreement. North Korea. The duty of silence, the isolation, and the poor nutrition demean the participants and turn them into zombies. What's more, leaving is forbidden, no matter how bad you feel. No, defenders argue, if you want to go you can go, no one's stopping you, it's just strongly discouraged. Above all, the participants themselves commit to staying until the end. I was intrigued but not put off by such discussions: I feel immune to sectarian indoctrination, I'm even curious about it. "Come and see," Christ said to those who had heard all sorts of contradictory rumors about him, and that still seems to me to be the best policy: come and see, with as little prejudice as possible, or at least with an awareness of whatever prejudices you have.

Zafu in Brittany

I've been married twice, and both times I made albums of family photos. Then when you separate, you never know where these albums will end up. The children look at them with nostalgia, because they show the times when they were little, when their parents loved each other like they should, when things still hadn't gone wrong. My first wife, Anne, and I spent the summer vacation in Brittany, at Pointe de l'Arcouest, where we rented a house that was marvelous but completely run-down because it was owned jointly and none of the co-owners saw why they, and not their brothers or sisters, should change a lightbulb. Facing Île-de-Bréhat, it had a superb view of the sea, which we reached by walking down a wooded path that was so steep and so wild that each summer it had to be cleared with a machete. Anne was incredibly pretty. She wore blue-and-white-striped jerseys and a bright yellow raincoat, I had unruly locks of hair and little round glasses. I would have liked to look mature, I looked like an adolescent. In the mornings we went to get crêpes at the village bakery, in the evenings we bought crabs down at the docks. Among the many photos of our two little boys, one in my album shows me on the beach with Gabriel, aged three or four, doing the canonical series of yoga postures called the sun salutation, and another shows Jean-Baptiste sitting on a zafu, laughing the happy laugh of a child. These photographs date the practices I'm discussing here, and attest that at the beginning of the 1990s I already had a zafu. I was already sitting on it, early in the mornings, taking pains to wake up before everyone else to observe my breathing and the flow of my thoughts. A zafu, if you don't know, is a round, compact Japanese cushion, specially designed to help you sit upright while meditating. Our boys liked to call this black zafu Zafu, as if it were a pet, a second dog—the first one being a mangy, one-eyed mongrel we called "the poor old guy," who lived somewhere in the neighborhood and came to see us every day. I know that these memories interest only Anne, the boys, and me, that we're the only four people in the world whom they can make smile, or cry, but too bad, too bad for you, reader, you'll have to put up with the fact that authors relate these kinds of things and don't delete them when they're rereading what they've written, as would only be reasonable, because they're precious, and because one reason to write is also to save them.

Tai chi on the mount

As I wrote in the questionnaire, I started to meditate thanks to tai chi. You know what tai chi is, I believe? Those very slow movements that people—often quite old—do in parks, dressed in padded Chinese jackets? Is it a dance? Gymnastics? A martial art? Originally it was a martial art, but unfortunately it's often taught as if this dimension didn't exist. I thank my lucky stars that I first ran across the Dojo de la Montagne, on Rue de la Montagne Sainte Geneviève, on the Left Bank in Paris, rather than one of those New Age groups that were springing up all around, where you were invited to open your chakras by burning incense sticks. Burning incense sticks wasn't the thing at the Dojo de la Montagne. The oldest karate dojo in Paris, it was established in the fifties by a pioneer called Henry Plée and headed, when I arrived, by his son, Pascal. Pascal got his white belt on his third birthday and has since trained a generation of karatekas, but with time, seeing that intensive training hurt the back, the knees, the joints, he started to look for more gentle, less arduous techniques, focusing less on force and more on flexibility. That's how he came to study tai chi under a Chinese master called Yang Jwing-Ming—*Dr.* Yang Jwing-Ming—who wasn't only a practitioner but also a very high-caliber researcher in the practically boundless field of what's known as the "internal" martial arts. I still have a half dozen of his books, which I studied fervently at the time. Because after a couple of months at the Dojo de la Montagne I was hooked, and stayed that way for almost ten years. Practically ten whole years, with three or four classes per week—not counting Dr. Yang's annual seminar—I spent immersed in the strange culture that is the dojo. More than dinners or parties, I've always appreciated this sort of get-together where you don't just meet to talk or *see each other*, as they say, but to do something together. No matter what: hiking, soccer, motorbiking. My ideal would have been to meet up with a few friends and play chamber music, say the viola in an amateur string quartet: you arrive at a member's place and exchange a few perfunctory words, then very quickly you unfold the stands, spread out the music, and pick up where you left off, at the sixteenth bar of the *andante con moto*. Unfortunately, I love music without being able either to read or play it. But I think that doing tai chi is much like singing or playing an instrument. It requires the same perseverance, the same blend of rigor and abandon, and I think with fondness of all the people of such different backgrounds and temperaments with whom I spent so many hours, practicing and perfecting infinitely slow movements the way a pianist practices and perfects the equivalent of this infinite slowness on the piano: the *larghissimo*. I was going to say that we all came for the same reason and were united by the same desire, but that's not quite it. There were two families at the Dojo de la Montagne: on the one hand the pounders, Pascal's close guard, made up of robust karatekas who, notwithstanding all the talk, were there to learn how to beat up their fellow men, and on the other those I'll call the spiritualists, and by that I don't mean the New Age chatterboxes who were quickly put off by the dojo's demanding routine, but people who were interested in Zen, in the Tao, in meditation. And the great thing was that under the double leadership of Pascal and Dr. Yang, these two families not only got along peacefully but also shared each other's interests. Very naturally, and while both groups would have been horrified if you'd told them this was where they were heading, the spiritualists like me found themselves doing karate *as well as* tai chi so as to make the tai chi they were doing more martial, while the pounders increasingly found themselves sitting motionless on little cushions and observing their breath.

It's complicated

Sitting motionless on a little cushion and observing your breath is what's called meditation. It's a practice that's becoming more and more widespread, and it would have been the sole subject of this book if life hadn't taken it, as you'll see, toward stormier terrain. Dr. Yang taught it with care. He was Chinese, he appreciated technique—bless his heart—he didn't rush things, and he considered meditation the apogee of the martial arts, but also a dangerous practice due to the powerful forces it awakens. He put us on guard against these dangers, which it seems to me I've never faced, either because I was never aware of them or more probably because I've never reached and never will reach the level at which they become a threat. As he didn't want us to go astray on the dangerous paths leading to the chasms within us, a bit like the way you give to novices a taste of the raptures they'll later experience, Dr. Yang taught us the rudiments of meditation by means of numerous diagrams, meridian pathways, normal breathing (Buddhist) and inverted breathing (Taoist), small and large circulation. And—as I just wrote on the page of the questionnaire dealing with my experience with meditation— what I know a bit about is the small circulation. After that I practiced with another master, Faeq Biria, who gained his profound knowledge of Iyengar yoga from the founder himself, B.K.S. Iyengar. Faeq Biria goes further than Dr. Yang, and maintains that to start meditating you need at least ten years of assiduous practice. You have to have opened the pelvic region, opened the shoulders, aligned the *bandhas*, aligned the *chakras*, and mastered all the techniques of *pranayama*, and only then does this grand, mysterious, transformative thing called meditation happen, and it happens on its own. Everything you did before was merely aimed at making it possible. Someone who shows up at an Iyengar yoga school and asks naively if, in addition to postures, it's also possible to do a bit of meditation is treated with indulgence, but at the same time like a bit of a nitwit. He's told nicely that there's as good as no difference between what the fashionable gurus and books on personal development call meditation and twiddling your thumbs: that without long preparatory work you can spend thousands of hours on a zafu focusing on your breath or the point between your eyebrows, but you could just as well be taking a nap.

It's simple

These two masters, both of whom I knew personally, are true, great masters, equally researchers and artists: I do not call their authority into question. However, from the height of my minute experience, I believe that you can gain access to meditation over a path that's less steep, a shorter path that's open to everyone, and that all the technique you need to take it can be learned in five minutes. It consists in sitting down for a while and remaining silent and motionless. Everything that happens inside you during the time you remain seated, silent and motionless, is meditation. I've often looked for a good definition—as simple, accurate, and all-encompassing as possible—and while there are others that I'll unpack as this story progresses, this one seems to be the best to start off with because it's the most concrete and the least intimidating. I repeat: meditation is everything that happens inside you during the time when you're seated, silent and motionless. Boredom is meditation. The pains in your knees, back, and neck are meditation. The rumbling of your stomach is meditation. The feeling that you're wasting your time with bogus spirituality is meditation. The telephone call that you prepare in your head and the desire to get up and make it are meditation. Resisting this desire is meditation—giving in to it isn't, though, of course. That's all. Nothing more. Anything more is too much. If you do that regularly, for ten minutes, twenty minutes, half an hour a day, then what happens during this time when you remain seated, silent and motionless, changes. Your posture changes. Your breathing changes.

Your thoughts change. All of that changes because in any case everything changes, but also because you're observing it. You don't do anything in meditation, the key thing is not to do anything, except observe. You observe the appearance of your thoughts, your emotions, your sensations in your field of consciousness. You observe their disappearance. You observe what buoys them up, their points of reference, their convergence lines. You observe their passing. You don't cling to them, you don't repel them. You follow the flow without letting yourself be carried away by it. As you do that, it's life itself that changes. At first you don't notice. You have the vague feeling that you're on the cusp of something. Little by little, it becomes clearer. You detach a little, just a little, from what you call yourself. A little is already a lot. It's already enormous. It's worth it. It's a journey. At the start of this journey, a Zen saying goes, the distant mountain looks like a mountain. As the journey unfolds, the mountain never stops changing. You no longer recognize it, it's replaced by a series of illusions, you no longer have any idea where you're heading. At the end of the journey it's a mountain once again, but it has nothing at all to do with what you saw from a distance, long ago, when you started the journey. It *really is* the mountain. You can finally see it. You've arrived. You're there.

You're there.

Meditating while drunk

We drank a lot during the summers at Pointe de l'Arcouest, and the friends who came to visit drank quite a lot as well. Less, however, than the writer Jean-François Revel, whom we'd run into at the supermarket in nearby Paimpol, pushing his cart full of wine bottles. Revel was a scowly, no-necked apoplectic, yet he wrote dazzling books full of lucidity and acerbic wit. I don't know anyone who knows as much about Marcel Proust as he did, or with a more accurate, Orwellian take on the totalitarianism and obscenity of leftist intellectuals, and I love the fact that this one man cultivated such diverse interests. I had no idea that thirty years later his marvelous anthology of French poetry would practically save my life. What I also didn't know was that he was Matthieu Ricard's father. At the time no one knew who Matthieu Ricard was, that he was the Dalai Lama's right-hand man or that he would become the best-known propagator of Buddhism and meditation in France—in a way that gets on my nerves a bit, because I have a problem with saffron robes and monks who tell you: "Religions are sectarian and specialized: what I'm teaching isn't a religion, it's simply the truth." Anyway, we drank a lot, we drank too much, so that even though I remained true to meditation, I often did it with a hangover or even completely drunk. It was while I was completely drunk that I practiced circulating the breath and energy, first up the back to the crown of my head, then down the front of my body (that's basically the small circulation), all with heaps of autosuggestion and amid a maelstrom of parasitic thoughts that I was not only not able to calm but that also struck me as just terrific. That was short-lived, of course. When you're drunk or stoned—I was often both—you think you're finding nuggets of gold, then you come down and realize they're lumps of turd. With age, I've mellowed out. I still like getting drunk, but I have less and less tolerance for alcohol. Now it takes me three or four days to get over a binge, whereas at Pointe de l'Arcouest I was up and drinking the very next night. Meditating while drunk is absurd, I agree, but at the time I persuaded myself that I was observing my drunken state. Because the interest of meditation—this could be a second definition—is that it awakens a sort of witness inside you, who monitors the whirlwind of thoughts without being swept away by them. You're nothing but chaos, confusion, a bundle of memories, fears, phantoms, and vain longings, but inside you someone calmer is looking on and making a report. Of course, alcohol and drugs turn this secret agent into a double agent who can't be trusted. Nevertheless, I didn't stop meditating, I've always more or less kept at it, and if I persist in writing this book—my own version of those personal development books that sell so well in the bookshops—it's to say what personal development books rarely do: that those who practice the martial arts, Zen, yoga, meditation, all the big, radiant, beneficial things I've sought all my life, are not necessarily wise or calm or serene, but sometimes—often, even—pathetically neurotic like me, and that that doesn't prevent them from, in Lenin's strong words, "working with the available material," that in fact you have to do just that, and that even if it doesn't get you anywhere, you're right to persist on this path.

In the clear?

I wrote these jaded lines two years after the incidents they relate, in a room in the Sainte-Anne Psychiatric Hospital, where between electroshocks I tried to keep my weary, roaming mind in check by patching together this story. However, on the night of January 7, 2015, lying on the narrow bed of my bungalow on an isolated farm in the Morvan region and waiting for dinnertime to arrive as a heavy rain pounded down on the soft black earth of the garden, I saw things in a less cruel light. At that time, even if I didn't see myself as calm, appeased, and serene—not entirely, not yet—at least I saw myself as someone who was no longer pathetically neurotic. For Freud, mental health is being able both to love and to work, and to my great surprise for almost ten years I'd been able to do both. If someone had told me when I was younger that that would be the case, I wouldn't have believed them. I didn't expect that much from life. The fact is, though, that one after the other, and without long or torturous periods of dryness, I had written four big books that many people had liked, and I thanked heaven each day for a marriage that made me happy. After so many years of sentimental drifting, I believed I had reached port, and that my love was sheltered from storms. I'm not crazy: I know full well that all love is endangered—that in any event everything is endangered— but from then on I imagined this danger as coming from the outside, and no longer from within me. Freud has a second definition of mental health, just as striking as the first: no longer prey to neurotic misery, but just to common unhappiness. Neurotic misery is a state we ourselves create in a horribly repetitive way, ordinary unhappiness one that life holds in store for us in ways that are as varied as they are unpredictable. You have cancer, or worse yet, one of your children has cancer, you lose your job and are plunged into poverty: ordinary unhappiness. I myself have been largely spared ordinary unhappiness: no great sorrows, no health or money problems, children who are making their way in life, and the rare privilege of having a career I love. As far as neurotic misery goes, though, I'm second to none. Without wanting to brag, I'm exceptionally good at turning a life replete with all it takes to be happy into a veritable hell. And I won't have anyone making light of this hell: it's real, terribly real. However, against all odds, it seems I've escaped it. In January 2015, it seems I can say

I'm *in the clear*. Of course, I'm careful not to get smug, I know it could be an illusion—but is an illusion that lasts ten years still an illusion? What makes this moment of my life so good? What's behind this progress? Psychoanalysis? Frankly I don't think so. I've spent almost twenty years on couches without any noticeable results. No, I think it's simply love. And maybe meditation. *Yoga, meditation*: I use these two words more or less interchangeably. I think that like love and writing, yoga and meditation will accompany, support, and carry me with them until I die. I view the last quarter of my life—because statistically, at almost sixty, that's the phase I'm entering—in line with Glenn Gould's maxim, which I've copied so often into so many successive notebooks: "The purpose of art is not the release of a momentary ejection of adrenaline but is, rather, the gradual, lifelong construction of a state of wonder and serenity."

Castles in the air

The gradual, lifelong construction of a state of wonder and serenity: it's pleasant to think of your life in these terms. Such thoughts are pleasant; they're thoughts of gratitude, harmonious thoughts, good thoughts. At the same time, I know myself, and I know inside and out the direction these thoughts will take me in, the smug images they'll waste no time evoking. As I near sixty, I imagine this better version of myself, this upgraded Emmanuel: serene and good-natured, with a center of gravity from which words with true weight resound—and not the "hollow sound" produced by bloated entrails, which Nietzsche talks about. A man who's made peace with his fearful, narcissistic little ego, whose books are ever more limpid and universal, and whose fame is universal as well, bidding his friends welcome under the pergola of his simple, lovely house on the Greek island of Patmos, nearing death without blinking in this eminent state of wonder and serenity that he spent his life constructing. Okay: laugh all you like. In fact, although I do my best not to spend too much time toying with such images, I don't spurn them either, the way a desert hermit spurns the temptations of the flesh. I would have at one time, when I was a guilt-ridden Christian. Today I say to myself: of course these are just flattering, narcissistic reveries, but is that such a bad thing? All told, they're rather innocent, and this ideal self of mine isn't as crummy as all that either. And above all, even if it's a little lame to take pleasure in them, it's even lamer to try to sweep them under the rug. Because the revolution—or one of the revolutions—of meditation is just that. Instead of looking askance at thoughts you're not so proud of, instead of trying to eradicate them, you stick to observing them without blowing them out of proportion. Because they exist, because they're there. Neither true nor false, neither good nor evil: mental micro events, bubbles on the surface of consciousness. When viewed in that way, they lose their sting and their control over you, without your even noticing it. Not judging your thoughts, any more than you judge your fellow humans, taking them for what they are, seeing them as they are—this is a third, and perhaps the most accurate, definition of meditation: seeing your thoughts as they are. Seeing things as they are.

Things as they are

Seeing things as they are: that's what *Vipassana* means. And *Things as They Are* is the title of a book on Buddhism written by my friend Hervé Clerc. I've already told Hervé's story in *The Kingdom*, but, as I have to struggle against my pretentious tendency to believe that my readers have read and remember my other books, I'll now tell it again a bit differently, starting with a quote from Pythagoras. When asked "Why is man on earth?" Pythagoras answered: "To observe the heavens." To observe the heavens? If that's true, most people don't know it. Most people believe they're on earth to find love, get rich, wield power, promote growth, or otherwise leave their mark on the sands of time. People who know they're here to observe the heavens are rare. If you're not one yourself, you can count yourself lucky to know one. It expands your horizons. I have that luck: I know Hervé, a peaceful, laconic, thoughtful guy who lives each moment as if it could be his last and who's always careful not to clutter up his life. Like Diogenes, he thinks it's better to drink from his hands than from a cup. When he travels, he tears out the pages of his books as he reads them to lighten his load. A journalist with the news agency Agence France-Presse, he's lived in Spain, the Netherlands, and Pakistan, and has always made a point of not letting his career get the upper hand, and of remaining, as he says, under the radar. Today he divides his time between Nice and Le Levron, a village in the Valais region of Switzerland, where he has an apartment in a chalet overlooking two valleys. It's a panorama of exceptional beauty, in front of which he's spent a lot of time meditating and written three books exploring what the mystics have said about ultimate reality, long designated by the code name God, which in his view no longer suits us. For thirty years now, Hervé and I have met up at Le Levron to walk on the mountain trails, talk a little, and be silent a lot. A local joke I like a lot goes like this: Three bumpkins sit on a bench. A cow goes by and the first bumpkin says, "That's Pierrot's cow." A quarter of an hour goes by, then the second one says: "No, it was Fernand's." Another quarter of an hour goes by, then the third one gets up and walks off, saying: "I've had enough of your bickering." And that's what our conversations are like, except we don't bicker. Our friendship is one my life's graces, and I think of his as well. It has known neither storms nor eclipses, and yet it's nourished by profound differences, and even by a major disagreement. Hervé thinks we're here not just to contemplate the sky, but also to find a way out of this confusion that is life on earth. He thinks that certain explorers found the way out and show us the way. Those explorers are Plato, Buddha, Meister Eckhart, Teresa of Ávila, and Patanjali—of whom I'll soon have more to say. And nothing, for Hervé, is more necessary or more urgent than reading their reports and examining the maps they drew up for us to follow them. To say it with Indian words—because no civilization has thought as much, as

deeply, or as accurately about these topics as the Indian—
the task, the only task, that a man of good sense must seek
to accomplish is to leave samsara, this wheel of change and
suffering we call the human condition, and gain access to
nirvana, where life is finally real, void of illusion, where
you see things as they are. That is yoga, Hervé says. Or
rather: that's what yoga is if you take it seriously, and not
just as a form of gymnastics.

Pasture hiking

I don't say the opposite, I rarely say the opposite of what
anyone says. But I'm not as certain that there is a way
out, or that the only goal in life is to look for it, or that
that's the only reason to do yoga. I waver, that's my nature.
One day I believe it, the next day I don't. I don't know
what's true, or if there is a truth. And even if I'm heading
toward the mountain, I don't think I'll reach the summit.
I'll never be one of those spiritual mountaineers we call
mystics. And it doesn't matter, because there's a middle
way between navigating the eternal snows and languishing
on the valley floor. It's what's called, sometimes disdain-
fully, pasture hiking. I'm a meditator on a pasture hike. I
like hiking in the mountain pastures, and when I do it's
like meditating. I try to blend my steps, my breathing, my
sensations, my perceptions, and my thoughts into one. And
that's also what pushes me, every morning or almost every
morning, to sit cross-legged on the zafu. I like it: it's as
simple as that. When I'm there, I feel like I'm in my place.

For this half hour I feel good, and I know from experience
that this feeling of well-being will become part of my day.
That it will make me a little more present, a little more
attentive to those around me. There are people who've had
experiences while meditating. Really strong ones, which
transported them outside of themselves or into a region
of themselves they never thought existed. Perhaps some
have even teleported, as Bismillah in Tiruvannamalai had
hoped to. Not me. I have sensed a certain peace, felt more
at ease with myself and others, but I've never experienced
anything out of the ordinary like rapture, a cessation of
thoughts, emptiness, illumination or even a premonition of
illumination, light at the end of the tunnel. Well, in fact
there was one time, at the Hotel Cornavin in Geneva: I'm
planning on talking about that when the time comes. For
now, however, as I grope to tell this story, I have no idea
when that time will be. Until then, pasture hiking suits me
just fine.

What we expect

But if that suits me fine, and if a mellow, regular routine is
enough for me, why did I sign up for this commando version of meditation? This brings me back to one of their four
simple, direct questions: What do I expect? My answer: an
impulse, a mild push that will give me the momentum to
pick up where I left off a couple of months ago. If I'd had to
say more, I could have added that the previous autumn I'd
published a book, *The Kingdom*, which had been a success,

that my ego had been flattered and I'd been in the lime-light around the clock, and that although that was all the more reason to meditate each morning, I hadn't been able to and I'd resigned myself to that fact. Meditation—fourth definition—consists in examining the person you really are, the magma we call an identity, and the person I really was at that moment was in no mood to meditate, that's all. The idea, then, now that the excitement had subsided, was to get back to my good habits. To get myself back on track thanks to this intensive training. There: that's the reason I can admit. But in saying that, I'm skirting the issue, and at one point I'll have to admit another, perhaps less avowable reason: if I'm here, it's to write a book.

The back-cover blurb

As I've discussed yoga and meditation in passing in my other books, one day a journalist came to interview me about these trendy subjects. Two things surprised me: first, the pleasure I felt in talking about them, and second, the ignorance of this young man who was otherwise both curi-ous and cultivated. He was astonished to discover that yoga is more than a kind of aerobics, and that meditation isn't just an esoteric curiosity. And when, taken by enthusiasm, I went on to discuss tai chi and the Chinese variants of these Indian practices, he started jotting down the words *yin* and *yang* in his notebook with stunned amazement, as if I were deciphering cuneiform characters. Even more surprisingly, I observed the same ignorance among many practitioners of yoga, and it struck me that it could be both a useful and a pleasant task to write a short, unpretentious book in a conversational tone, an upbeat, subtle little book explaining the topic from my own experience—the experience of an apprentice, needless to say, and not of a master. I even went as far as writing a short pitch for the book in the form of a back-cover blurb. It's very strange for me to copy it down now, seeing as how the book has changed so much from what I thought it would be. But here it is:

> What I call yoga isn't just the beneficial gymnastics so many of us practice, but rather a group of disciplines aimed at broadening and unifying the mind. Yoga tells us that we are something other than our confused, little, fearful, and fragmented ego, and that we can have access to this other thing. It's a path. Others have taken it before us and shown us the way. If what they say is true, it's well worth embarking on the journey ourselves.

A pleasant task, yes, and a useful one. And what's more, I thought eagerly, a tremendous number of people do yoga today, a tremendous number of people would be happy to know more about what they're doing when they do it: this book could sell like hotcakes.

The welcome speech

Before we stop talking for ten days, there's a welcome speech about the measures we agree to abide by during the session. It's the nice young man who gives it. He does it in a laid-back way, without assuming the authority of a master. He and the two guys at his side are simply practitioners who, after having done one, two, or three sessions like ours, chose to come back as helpers. They meditate as well, of course, everyone does, but instead of resting between the sessions they help with the cooking, cleaning, and various organizational tasks; in a word, they keep the place running. It's what's known as karma yoga, or yoga of action or service: a humble and effective way of giving back the benefits you've received. "It might surprise you," says the nice young man, "but in the twenty years that Vipassana has existed in France we've got a fair bit of hindsight, and going by the statistics, a quarter of you will come back as helpers. Some of you will yourselves give this speech to the new arrivals, and not too long from now, either." After that a reminder of our various commitments: not to leave the enclosure, and within the enclosure, which includes a bit of forest, to keep to the fenced paths; to respect the separation between the area reserved for the men and the area reserved for the women; to respect the silence; not to communicate with the outside world or among ourselves, even nonverbally; to avoid exchanging glances as much as possible; in case problems arise, to speak with the teacher and with him only; and finally, the key point, to stay until the end.

"There's still time to leave," says the nice young man, and his smiling face grows stern. "If you have doubts, if you're not sure you'll respect these commitments, we ask that you leave now. No one will blame you. You won't harm yourself or anyone else. You can come back when you feel ready. Leaving now isn't cowardly. On the contrary, it's good. It proves that you appreciate the situation, it's the right thing to do. But if for some reason you decide to leave midsession you'll throw the others off, and above all you'll put yourself in danger. What happens during a Vipassana session is very serious. We work with very powerful psychic energies; something like that can disrupt the whole process. You might have a hard time over the next ten days. You might get disoriented or feel lost, you might cry or be afraid, or think you were wrong to come. That's possible. Many reactions are possible, there's no way of telling what can happen. If things go wrong, the teachers are here to help. But you must respect the vow you make this evening: *Whatever happens, I will remain until the end.* So please, think about it. And after you've thought about it, leave if you must. But if you decide to stay, stay."

There follows a moment of silence, longer than the one at a wedding after the pro forma question of whether anyone sees any reason that the couple shouldn't be married. No one asks: Still, if I want to go, will I be able to? You won't stop me? No doubt the answer would be: The problem isn't whether you'll be stopped or not—you *must not* leave. Like in the Balkan country where politicians were subject to incessant attacks and finally a law was passed, stipulating "Shooting the finance minister, fifteen years in prison. Shooting the interior minister, twenty years. Shooting the chamberlain, ten years. *It is forbidden to shoot the prime minister.*"

No one gets up. No one leaves. Little do I know that, four days later, I'll be the first one to go.

Playing the game

The Noble Silence has begun. The helpers wheel around metal carts with huge platters of rice and boiled vegetables, which you can season with soy sauce, brewer's yeast, or gomashio. Everyone takes a bowl or a plate, which they don't wash after using but simply place in a plastic tub that the helpers take away. With material constraints reduced to a minimum, there is nothing, absolutely nothing to do other than be silent and turn your gaze inward. Other people's gazes are avoided. You stare at your plate, you eat very slowly, chewing for a very long time—a practice by which you can recognize the food control freaks, whose ranks I've been trying to join for years without much success. Once the meal is done, we go to bed early. Eyes downward, everyone goes back to their bungalow or dormitory. At 8 p.m. I'm in bed. With no book, nothing to do, and of course not the slightest desire to go to sleep, I watch the block of night framed in the window across from me. I look at the Gemini statue that I've placed on the empty shelf like it's a little altar. What I'd like to do, in fact, is to write down as faithfully as I can the speech given by the nice young man, and my impressions of the evening. Am I right in playing the game? In not having slipped a notebook into my bag? Yes: that would have been to turn this experience into some sort of report. At the same time, it'd be ridiculous to lie: what I'm doing here *is* a report. Or let's say: it's *also* a report. I'm under cover. I came to look for material for my book, and whether I take notes or not won't change a thing, because what deserves to be remembered will be remembered. But in fact, that's not the question. The question—and this isn't the first time I'm asking it—is whether there's an incompatibility, or even a contradiction, between the practice of meditation and my trade, which is to write. Over the next ten days, will I watch my thoughts go by without becoming attached to them, or will I instead try to hold on to them, which is the exact opposite of meditation? Will I spend the whole time taking mental notes? Will the meditator be observing the writer, or the writer observing the meditator? It's a big, big topic, and it gnaws at me until I fall asleep.

Strategic depth

In anticipation of life without a phone, I bought a big alarm clock from an Indian bazaar on Rue du Faubourg Saint-Denis—the most basic, cheapest kind, the kind that ticks. I set it for quarter past four, but at quarter past four I've been awake for ages, in fact I've hardly slept. When Charles de Foucauld woke up in the night, no matter what time it was, he made it a principle to get up and consider that the day had begun—a radical way of treating insomnia. Without always having the courage, I try to do the same. In Paris I get up before dawn and go to my study, without turning on a light or making a sound. I like to be the only one awake as the rest of the house sleeps, above all in the winter when it's still dark and the heating accentuates the drowsiness, sitting on the zafu and observing my breathing and what's going through my mind. This transition between sleeping and waking lasts about half an hour, after which my body needs to move. Tenuous at first, the movements gain in scope and gradually become asanas, as yoga postures are called. I've taken a lot of courses in the past, now I practice alone, early in the morning, as I please. I do the postures I want, as I want, as they progress and change into others. On good days you feel like an animal stretching. On less good days you take refuge in routine, set patterns and preferences—it's better than nothing. Depending on how you feel, there are static days and dynamic days, days when you sit and days when you stand. The advantage of taking classes is that there's someone to correct you, the advantage of practicing alone is that you learn to correct yourself, and to listen to what your body is telling you. The body has three hundred joints. The blood circulates through more than sixty thousand miles of arteries, veins, and capillaries. There are forty-six miles of nerves. Unfolded, the surface of the lungs would cover a soccer field. Little by little, yoga aims to become acquainted with all of this. To fill it all with consciousness, energy, and the consciousness of energy. When you sign up for your first class, that's the last thing you expect. You expect to become healthier and calmer. You expect to gain a little strategic depth—as the military top brass call the potential retreat zone in case of a border attack. Germany, whose territory is encircled, has very little, whereas Russia has a lot—which goes a long way to explaining the outcome of the Second World War. And this image translates well on an individual level. Faced with outward aggression, people have more or less ability to fall back into themselves, more or less strategic depth. Better health, more calm, strategic depth: all of this you get when you do yoga. But such benefits are only spillovers, collateral benefits. Even if you're not aware of it, and even if like me you stick to easy paths and pasture hikes, you're on your way to somewhere else.

The gong

No yoga last night, no meditation: I stay in bed, curled up, somewhat anxious, waiting for the alarm to ring. It rings, I turn it off. My eyes riveted on the dial, I watch the second hand move in jerks: it's become rare to see an old-style, nondigital mechanism in movement. Twenty past four: I give myself five more minutes. But before those five minutes are up, a sound emerges from the night, extraordinarily grave, extraordinarily full, extraordinarily deep. You'd think a very heavy stone had fallen into the thick water of a black lake and was tracing slow circles. You'd think that those circles would never stop spreading, that their vibrations would continue endlessly. They hypnotize me. I feel like they'll cover me, never stop covering me. Then they start to ebb. There's no telling exactly when this ebb started, it's like when inhaling comes to an end and becomes exhaling. The sound fades gradually, but in fading it grows even graver, deeper. In certain yoga classes you start by chanting the sound *Om*, which is the primordial sound in Hinduism, a mantra reduced to its simplest expression. For a long time it annoyed me, as if I were being asked to sing hymns. However, it must be said that when the vibration moves your whole body, it has a powerful effect. The vibration of the gong is the instrumental equivalent, and I now realize that it's been hit for a second time, that the lake of sound in which I've been swimming for almost a minute came from a single stroke of the mallet. So I get up, dress quickly, and pull up the blind. White-globed lampposts line the path that leads through the garden. Under the rain, silhouettes leave their bungalows and walk slowly toward the hall. You'd think we were in a zombie film.

The hall

The ground is black and muddy, I'm glad I brought good shoes. We're all wearing beanies, it's a bit like in a mountain hut just before dawn when everyone's getting ready to head out, except that in a mountain hut you drink tea or coffee from thermoses and eat cereal bars, and above all you look at one another, exchange a few words, or make funny faces to show how hard it was to get out of your sleeping bag. Not here. We don't look at one another. We look down, or up at the sky, which is starless and as black as the earth. After the third stroke, the gong has stopped. At the entrance to the hall, the nice young man starts calling out our names: each name corresponds to the number of a place in the hall, and we'll keep these places for the entire session. When your name is called, you leave your parka and shoes in the cloakroom, take cushions and blankets from the shelves, and carry them into the hall. It's a huge hall, divided in half by an empty space ten or twelve feet across. On the left, us, the men, on the right, the women,

who come in through a door on the opposite side. Each
space comprises one flat cushion measuring roughly thirty
inches a side. Later I'd count them all: six per row, ten
rows, multiplied by two, meaning there were one hundred
and twenty of us. The cushions are basic, and solid blue.
So are the zafus, which everyone will pile as high as they
need to sit up straight. But while the men's blankets are
blue, the women's are white. They're soft and warm, it's a
pleasure to wrap yourself in one—but there's little need
because like my room, the hall is perfectly heated. At the
far end of the hall there's a platform in front of each group.
A man sits cross-legged and wrapped in a blue blanket in
front of the men, a woman draped in a white blanket sits
in front of the women. The man is thin, with a protruding
Adam's apple and a calm face. The woman has short white
hair, but I can only see her from a distance because my
place is on the far side of the men's section. Pretty soon, in
any case, I'll lose all interest in the women's section. One
after the other, my neighbors colonize the space marked out
by their square cushions, which play the same role as the
mat in yoga classes: all movements must take place inside
this space, without ever crossing the border or encroach-
ing on the space of the next person. There's something
very seductive in the idea that one can be happy within a
perimeter of twenty-four by sixty-eight inches. You could
imagine that if you were in prison, for example, all you'd
need to do would be to spread out a yoga mat to assert
a sort of freedom in the suffocation of your cell. One of
my neighbors grabs his ass cheeks with both hands and
spreads them apart to distribute the muscles of his pelvic

floor on the cushion—a gesture that can seem strange to the uninitiated, but by which you can unfailingly recognize a practitioner of Iyengar yoga. He does it unceremoniously and so do I, marking my obedience before taking up the posture.

The posture

I said it was very simple to meditate, that it boils down to sitting for a moment, silent and motionless. Right away I have to add that there are all kinds of ways of sitting: cross-legged, the half lotus, the lotus, the *seiza* posture— Japanese-style with your legs folded underneath you—or on a chair if you're not so flexible . . . All of these are fine, so long as they provide a minimum of comfort and allow you to sit upright, even if it means using cushions. Because you have to sit upright. As straight as you can. Stretching your spine upward, as if you wanted to push on the ceiling with the top of your head. At the same time you must keep rooted, making sure that the bottom of your spine and pelvis are pulled downward. The top of the spine pushes toward the sky, the bottom pulls toward the earth. Stretched in this way, the spine arches, grows longer, and the spaces between the vertebrae widen. You accompany the spine as it rises from the sacrum to the occiput. You observe its curves, and what happens when you try to invert them, protruding the concave bits and pulling in the convex bits. As I stretch I feel—and hear—one of my vertebrae cracking. It's a pleasant sound, and the sensation that accompanies it is pleasant and encouraging as well. There's no doubting that it's good for you. Stretching your spine like that is a full-time occupation. But even as you do it you have to carry out another full-time occupation, which consists in relaxing: your face, your shoulders, your stomach, your hands, everything you can relax, and that's a lot—in fact, it's limitless. When you take stock of everything that's tense, you realize that this, too, is a full-time occupation. Stretching your spine as much as you can while relaxing everything else makes two full-time occupations to do at the same time. Well, at the start, *almost* at the same time. Let's say in parallel, as if you were leading two horses under the same yoke, both of whom want to head off in different directions. In fact, that's the original meaning of the word *yoga*: harnessing two horses or buffaloes under one yoke. You pass from one to the other, then back. And when you try to pay attention to what you're doing, even a little—which is the point of the whole exercise—there's no time to be bored. The more demanding the posture becomes, the more you start to like it. It's a pleasure to settle into it each day, to come back to it at a given time. To hold it for longer and longer. To feel when it starts to sag. Then you correct and refine it, appreciating more and more the equilibria that make it up. Some days it's a pleasure, others it's unbearable. Nothing works. Your whole body protests and resists your stillness, and you no longer perceive a single one of the subtle, tense equilibria it was so enjoyable to observe. At such times the best thing would be to pay attention to this rebellion, this antipathy, this disgust. If you did, they'd become part of the meditation. But most often when you feel them, instead of paying attention you hurry to get things over with. You get up, go read your mail. Next time.

Rules for experiments

Everyone is silent, except for the guy to my right who sat down after me and is making a huge racket. Clearing his throat, making little sounds with his mouth, breathing heavily—and, at least as far as his breathing is concerned, I get the feeling that he's doing it on purpose, that he thinks that's how it's done and that it doesn't bother him at all to be the only one doing it. Ten days next to this guy would be like sharing a dorm with someone who snores or smells bad: I don't know how I'm going to last. Furtively, I open my eyes and sneak a quick look to my right, and I'm not surprised to see it's the little guy with the jacquard sweater and goatee who already got on my nerves way back when we were still talking, with his discourse on letting go. Letting go, living in the present moment: I know the drill, and even if the idea seems right to me, I've noticed that like libertarianism, it's often defended by real obsessives. And I've noticed that this little guy, who's so eager to hold out his serenity as an example, performs any task—be it picking up a bowl or pouring wheat germ on his soup—with twice as many gestures as necessary. Ever since I saw him yesterday evening, he's reminded me of someone. And now, suddenly, I remember who: Mr. Ribotton, my eighth-grade science teacher. Really marvelous teachers who awaken their pupils' understanding do exist. They're rare, and you can count yourself terrifically lucky if you meet a single one when you're going to school. But you also meet some real wackos, and Mr. Ribotton's wackiness came out in a very particular way. Science class involves experiments, one of the main ones being dissecting frogs. To prepare us, Mr. Ribotton had worked out a series of "rules for experiments," whose importance he spent the entire first class stressing, and which he started dictating to us as early as the second. These rules were so detailed, so abundant, and took into account so many situations that could arise during experiments that the explanation continued through the third, fourth, and fifth classes, and the first test of the semester wasn't about the class itself, but about his rules for experiments. Mr. Ribotton was disappointed by our results: we hadn't really got the gist of his rules. These then had to be revised, broadened, completed. Dictated again, copied again. Our notebooks swelled with the rules for experiments, which increasingly came to resemble terms and conditions you have to acknowledge having read and understood, although they're a thousand pages long and no one ever reads them. We spent the entire year like that, copying, studying, and being tested on these ever-expanding rules for experiments, without ever doing a single one of the experiments they so rigorously set out. Mr. Ribotton must have passed away long ago, but I get the feeling his reincarnation is right here beside me, and I think to myself that meditating for ten days beside Mr. Ribotton, exposed to his noisy breathing and manic shuddering, will be no picnic. But no sooner have I thought this

than I think something else, namely that having me beside
you is probably no picnic either, and that the spirit of meditation consists precisely in considering Mr. Ribotton's presence beside me as a blessing: not as a cause for annoyance
or scornful irony, but as an occasion for benevolence and
equanimity. Because another definition of meditation—
I think we're at number five—is to consent to, and not run
away from, things that annoy you. To delve deeper into the
annoyance, to work as much with what annoys you as you
do with your breath. It's also—sixth definition—learning
not to judge, in any case to judge less, a little less. To give
up any sense of preeminence, which is both a moral fault
and a philosophical mistake. In the words of one Buddhist
sutra I love to the point of having quoted it twice already in
my books: "A man who judges himself superior, inferior, *or
even equal* to another does not understand reality."

The voice

We're now all seated. You can feel the expectation in the air. Each slot of meditation lasts two hours, and I wonder how I'm going to sit motionless for that long. Normally my limit is twenty minutes, half an hour. I wait for the man or the woman on the platform to speak and—at least for starters—guide us. No matter how well I understood what the nice young man said to us yesterday evening, no matter how much I've resolved to leave my critical sense in the cloakroom over the next ten days, I'm afraid this will be one of those benign, pious voices that exasperate me, those voices of priests of all persuasions—and New Age priests are the worst of all. Despite whatever good resolutions I may have made—*A man who judges himself superior, inferior,* . . . et cetera—I know I'll have a hard time putting up with that. What suddenly emerges from the silence, however, is a deep, cavernous voice, a voice from the depths of the ages or the oceans, which starts very slowly to intone something that must be a prayer, or an invocation, I suppose in Sanskrit—in fact, I'll find out later, it's in Pali. I understand that it's a recording, and that this cavernous voice must be that of the late S. N. Goenka, the Burmese-born master who is to the Vipassana method what B.K.S. Iyengar is to the method of yoga that bears his name. The prayer lasts a long time, a very long time. Then, after a very long silence, the master starts to talk in English, English with an Indian accent, the English of Peter Sellers in *The Party*, and what he says is translated into French—also a recording—in a clear, sonorous male voice. There's nothing you can say against a voice like that; I accept it straightaway.

"Inhale, exhale"

"Inhale, exhale," says the voice of S. N. Goenka in English.

"Inhale, exhale," the interpreter translates into French.

"Feel the air entering your nostrils, the air leaving your nostrils.

"Breathe calmly, without trying to control your breathing.

"Inhale, exhale: let the cycles take place naturally.

"Don't try to control. Don't try to guide.

"Just observe.

"Observe what happens. Observe the sensations.

"The sensations inside your nostrils.

"At the start you may think you can't feel sensations

inside your nostrils, but there are sensations all the time, in each millimeter of your body. On the surface of your skin, inside your body.

"In the zones where the inside and outside of your body meet.

"Do you feel a sensation of heat inside your nostrils? A sensation of cold? Do you feel like scratching yourself? Do you want to blow your nose?

"Do not give in to these urges. Observe them.

"Consider these urges as sensations. There are pleasant sensations and unpleasant sensations. We all seek pleasant sensations and avoid unpleasant sensations. The urge to scratch yourself is an unpleasant sensation. Observe the displeasure it causes you. Don't try to change anything. This unpleasant sensation is the reality of the moment, you are here to observe it. Just to observe it.

"Maybe for a moment you haven't been following your breathing. Maybe you're no longer paying attention to your sensations.

"Come back to them. Come back to your sensations, gently, diligently, with perseverance.

"Bring your mind back to your breathing, inside your nostrils.

"Bring your mind back to the present.

"The present is your breathing.

"Inhale, exhale."

The Bardo

According to Tibetan tradition, the days that follow death are far more crucial than the ones leading up to it. Those who have just died enter a dark, intermediary domain, a psychic labyrinth that can lead either to liberation from samsara—a.k.a. the worldly condition—or to a new, more or less favorable incarnation, or straight to hell. This twilight zone, which everyone must cross when they're dead, is called the Bardo. The Tibetans mapped it out with great precision: deceptive crossroads, landslides, packs of wild dogs, paths leading nowhere, light at the end of the tunnel . . . This guide to the Bardo, known as the *Bardo Thodol* or *Tibetan Book of the Dead*, is read to the dead for the three days that follow their death, to accompany them on their journey. I can well imagine S. N. Goenka performing this ritual. It strikes me that if I had just died, with my body lying in my coffin and my soul wandering in the Bardo, it would reassure me to hear him murmuring in my ear in an incomprehensible language that's as old as humanity, with his cavernous, peaceful, pensive, marvelously even voice, whose tempo I'm starting to grow accustomed to, the way you grow accustomed to Indian music. Rather than following a melody that unfolds in a linear way at a given tempo, Indian melodic modes, or ragas, stretch out infinitely, plunging you into a stillness that radiates in all directions, so that while you never know how far you are along, at the same time you're always in the center. The intervals between S. N. Goenka's sentences have now become so long that I'm sure each one must be the last, and then, since it isn't the last, that S. N. Goenka, or the person whose avatar he is, will continue to guide us right up to the gates of samsara. Lulled by S. N. Goenka's voice, we feel safe, ready to venture into the Bardo or the depths of ourselves, which is probably the same thing. Bewitched by S. N. Goenka's voice, the little monkeys that swing incessantly from branch to branch and that represent, in Buddhist imagery, the agitation and dispersal of the mind calm down and sit obediently at his feet. And then S. N. Goenka and his interpreter finally fall silent. We must accept that the last sentence was the last, and that we're on our own.

Paying attention

Seventh definition of meditation: paying attention. The philosopher and mystic Simone Weil said that that's the real point of studying: not to learn things—we already know enough—but to hone our skill at paying attention. The East knows more about this than the West. The East has established techniques, identified aids. Practitioners can help themselves freely from this stock. Some silently repeat a mantra. Others meditate to a Zen koan, those enigmatic, luminous phrases that a master gives to his disciple to ruminate on over a period of years: "What was your face like before you had one? Before your parents were born?" "What is the sound of one hand clapping?" With time, such questions are supposed to cause a sort of mental short circuit: at some point the fuse blows, discursive thought is extinguished, it's satori—the Japanese name for enlightenment. You can also watch the flame of a candle, following its tiniest movements, connecting your brain with the flame until you *become* the flame. Or you can sit in front of an object, no matter what it is, say my little Gemini statue, look at it as attentively as possible, and then close your eyes and attempt to visualize it, trying to reconstitute behind your eyelids, as precisely as possible, the contours that just instants ago traveled from your open eyes to your brain via the optic nerve. Having formed this mental image, you open your eyes after a moment and come back to the real image as it imprints on your retina, soaking it up as best you can and then closing your eyes again to further define the mental image. You discover that, on the inside of your eyelids as well as in the shape of a small statue, albeit simple, there is infinity. All of these techniques have their merits, there's something for everyone. But the most widespread, the most universal, remains paying attention to your breathing. It was in following the thread of his breath that the Buddha realized "the world, the arising of the world, the cessation of the world and the path leading to the cessation of the world"; in other words, he reached nirvana. Of all physical phenomena, breathing is the most accessible to consciousness. Try focusing on your digestion, or the circulation of your blood: I'm not saying these can't also be supports for meditation, in fact I'm sure they can. I'm just saying it's not something for beginners like you and me. Breathing is something we always have access to, since we never stop breathing. We can learn to guide it. By practicing tai chi, then yoga, I learned rudimentary elements of very subtle techniques: the lesser circulation, pranayama. But that's not what we're being asked to do here. What we're being asked to do here is something else, the very opposite, even. And, as Captain Haddock of the Tintin series says: "It's both very simple and very complicated." On the face of it, you'd think that breathing normally would be easier than guiding your breath along meridians. In fact, it's more complicated. Doing nothing specific sounds simple, but it's much more complicated than doing something specific, even something difficult. As for observing your breathing without it being changed by your observing it, it's not difficult, it's impossible. It's impossible, but we try. That's what we're here for.

My friends the nostrils

The air enters my nostrils. I observe it as it enters. The air leaves my nostrils. I observe it as it leaves. It's calm, regular. I observe how it brushes against the inside of my nasal cavity. It's light, delicate. Nostrils have a large number of nerves, so there's plenty to pay attention to. There's always something happening there. You can meditate for two hours on your nostrils without getting bored. This session is off to a good start: my nostrils are my best friends. Once you've left the entrance and delved a little deeper into the cavities, they widen into huge caverns. The more you explore them, the farther you move along their walls, the bigger they get, and the more you feel: prickling, bristling, tingling. Pulsing, even: yes, a pulsing feeling that just about obscures all the rest. Something's pulsing. I observe this something. I identify with this pulsing. It's not at all unpleasant, observing it isn't unpleasant either. It's good. It's good, except that my posture has slumped. Sagged. I have to straighten out, without ceasing to pay attention to my breath as it enters my nostrils or the pulsing at the back of my nasal cavity. I stretch my spine, thrusting the top of my head skyward. It's a lot to do all at the same time, and my mind takes advantage of this congestion to slip away. My mind never stops slipping away. It slips away from the now, from the real—which is the same thing, because only what is now is real. The Tibetan master Chögyam Trungpa used to say that we dedicate 20 percent of our cerebral activity to the present. As for the remaining 80 percent, with some people it's focused on the past, with others on the future. I, for one, spend a lot of time thinking about the future and not much about the past. Nostalgia is foreign to me. One could see that as the mark of a confident, optimistic, forward-looking person. But I fear that with me it's more the mark of an obsessive, because while everyone knows you can't change the past, you can always hold to the illusion that you can control the future. To keep myself from slipping down that slope, I often repeat to myself the great Jewish maxim "You want to make God laugh? Tell him about your projects." But that doesn't stop me from continuing to make him laugh. When God wants to lift his mood and have a good laugh, I'm sure he looks over at me, sitting on my zafu, focusing on my breathing and the inside of my nostrils while thinking about my upbeat, subtle little book on yoga. Its format, its chapters, its subheadings. I'm already thinking up sentences, wondering how many definitions of meditation I've got now, and it's at this moment I realize that my thoughts have got the better of me: past, present, Chögyam Trungpa, tell God about your projects, my next book, what will be in it, how successful it will be . . . Time to come back to my nostrils. Time to come back to the air as it enters my nostrils. Inhale, exhale. The air is a little cooler when it enters, a little warmer when it leaves, after the long path it's taken inside me. Outside. Inside. When is it still outside, when is it already inside? Eighth possible definition of meditation: observing the points of contact between what is oneself and what is not oneself. Between the inside and the outside, the interior and the exterior.

The Brothers Térieur

Mr. and Mrs. Térieur have two boys, twins. What did they name them?

Alex and Alan.

I love that joke. In French, *Alex Térieur* sounds like "on the outside," and *Alan Térieur* sounds like "on the inside." And with every book I write, there's always a moment when I think it could be called *The Brothers Térieur*. Because whatever I do, I wonder if in doing it I'm more on Alan's terrain or on Alex's. When I research a magazine piece about the Calais Jungle refugee camp, it's Alex who goes there. If it's a Vipassana session in the Morvan region, it's Alan. Alex does fieldwork, Alan observes his breathing on a zafu. Alex Térieur is yang, Alan Térieur is yin. Both of them breathe. But then who does what? Who inhales? Who exhales?

Exhaling

All my life I've had this symptom. Inhaling is easy for
me. Full, regular. My chest swells, it's as if I could fill it
forever. Only there comes a moment when this huge inhalation has to be exhaled, and this exhalation, by contrast,
is pinched, cramped. It peters out. From the diaphragm
to the lower abdomen, everything it should relax, it con-
tracts, compresses, oppresses. It's as if it were caught in a
bottleneck, a knot under my chest, like in a garden hose.
I've long wondered if this knot is physical or mental. A hose,
or my unconscious? The doctors prescribed little pills to
treat acid reflux, which is common among people who suffer from anxiety. These pills have no effect on the thing
that I believe constitutes my identity, and that yoga is better suited to deal with. Because inhaling, yoga tells us, is
taking, conquering, appropriating, with which I have no
problem at all. In fact, I can't do anything else, and my
chest cavity is the measure of my appetite. Exhaling is different. It's giving rather than taking, returning rather than
keeping. It's letting go. On this point as on others, Hervé is
my exact opposite. Exhaling is his strong point. He wants
nothing better than to lighten himself. We're all passing
through life, but he's aware of it. He doesn't settle in, he
acts like a tenant, or even a subtenant, whereas I have the
proprietor's instinct to spread out my possessions and "grow
and prosper" like the biblical patriarchs. My natural pro-
pensity is to grow, his is to diminish. I aspire to the light,
he to the darkness. I seek the sunny side of the hill, he the
shady side. Two ways of being, two kinds of men, and this

difference in our characters is the basis of our friendship: a yang man, a yin man, a man who inhales, a man who exhales. At the end of the day, exhaling is breathing your last, giving up the ghost. The anxiety lodged in my chest is nothing but the fear of death, and the work cut out for me in my remaining years, I think, is just that: learning to exhale.

Patanjali at the Café de l'Église

There's a canonical text on yoga dating somewhere from the third century BCE to the second century AD, no one's really sure, attributed to Patanjali, who's also believed to have been a grammarian. It's a thin collection of sutras—laconic, somewhat opaque aphorisms, which never talk about yoga in the sense that we understand it, as a physical discipline. Yoga as we understand it must already have existed in those times, because Plutarch tells us that when Alexander the Great's soldiers arrived on the Ganges plain, they were astonished to discover people they called gymnosophists, who contorted themselves to acquire wisdom—in other words, yogis. But Patanjali isn't interested in these contortionists. The only posture he knows is the lotus, completely immobile. In anticipation of the book on yoga and meditation I was hoping to write, which was to be called *Exhaling*, for reasons you now know, every

morning in the winter of 2015 I went to read Patanjali at
the Café de l'Église on Paris's Place Franz Liszt. There I
compared several translations and jotted down ideas in a
notebook dedicated to his writings. Apart from being instructive, this occupation gave me a gratifying and perhaps
unduly flattering idea of myself. Today, now that my life
has gone off the rails, I think back to those mornings at the
Café de l'Église with a blend of fondness, incredulity, and
bitter irony. I was full of myself. I was happy. I believed it
would last. Like Hervé, and like all Indian thinkers since
the Upanishads, Patanjali is interested only in one question: Is there a way out of this thing we call the human condition, samsara? Can we reprogram? Any other questions or
concerns he considers pointless: "Aside from this, nothing
is worth knowing." The good news is that—still according
to Patanjali and Hervé—the answer is yes, there is a way
out. We can reprogram. It's not easy, in fact it's the work of
one or several lifetimes, but it is possible, and it's what yoga
aims to achieve. It's a technique that involves going beyond
consciousness by observing consciousness. Patanjali is an
unrivaled observer, he knows the unconscious at least as
well as Freud does, and he sets out his discoveries in the
Indian way, that is, with lists: the six *darsanas* (categories of
Brahman thinking: yoga is one), the three *gunas* (attributes
of consciousness), the five *yamas* (necessary abstinences),
the five *niyamas* (equally necessary disciplines), the five
matrices of the *chitta vritti* (fluctuations of consciousness),
the eight limbs of the *ashtanga* (or the tree of yoga) . . . The
Indians love lists, infinite classifications that strike us as
arbitrary. It's their way of grasping the universe, whereas

we favor chronology, which is completely foreign to them. Patanjali's lists and classifications of mental and spiritual phenomena are fascinating, and deserve to be studied in detail. I spent many hours doing just that at the Café de l'Église in preparation for my book on meditation and yoga. Now, for a condensed definition of yoga and a ninth—royal—definition of meditation, the four Sanskrit words that form the second verse of the *Yoga Sutras*: "Yogas chitta vritti nirodha."

"Yogas chitta vritti nirodha"

Yogas: okay, this is yoga—the thing we're defining.
Chitta: the mental, the field of mental and psychic activity.
Vritti: the fluctuations of consciousness, the waves on the surface of consciousness.
Nirodha: cessation, extinction, stabilization.

Now you know everything: yoga is the cessation of the fluctuations of the mind.

Nirodha is open to interpretation. Cessation or stabilization? Extinction or control? Is it a question of stopping the endless hurly-burly of our thoughts once and for all, or, more modestly, of calming them, slowing them down, taming them? Patanjali is a maximalist. His sole goal—and according to him the goal of all people of good sense—is to reach nirvana, not to make the stay in samsara a bit more comfortable. Yoga is a war machine against the vritti, that is, the movements of the mind: the ripples and breakers, swells and surges, currents and undercurrents, gusts and squalls, that disturb the surface of consciousness. The parasitic thoughts and incessant chatter that prevent us from seeing things as they are: vipassana. Starting with very concrete work on the body and breathing, yoga aims first of all to calm the vritti, then to rarefy them, and finally to make them disappear. The mind, then, becomes (it seems) as clear and transparent as a mountain lake. Rid of the foam of our fears, reactions, and incessant commentary, it no longer reflects anything but the real. That's what's called deliverance, illumination, satori, nirvana. But Patanjali's a high mountain guide, and we're not obliged to follow him right up to the summit. As I've said, I'm happy with pasture hiking, and I think it's already a lot if meditation can help you gain a little mental stability and strategic depth, and if you can calm the vritti just a bit, just a tiny bit. And the technique for calming the vritti, the little monkeys that swing incessantly from branch to branch, dizzying and exhausting us, is first, to observe your breathing, second, to observe your sensations, and third, to observe your thoughts. Another definition of meditation: to calm the vritti, you observe the vritti.

Vritti

How long have I been sitting on my zafu? Less than two hours, certainly, maybe an hour and a half. Physically I'm doing all right, I'm holding out. I'm breathing calmly, it's even quite pleasant. But no matter how calmly I breathe while exploring the back of my nostrils, the little merry-go-round keeps turning. It turns all the time, you hardly notice it, but as you meditate you watch it turn. You're a little more aware of it, so you've made progress. Which vritti have rippled the surface of my consciousness since S. N. Goenka finished his raga? Well, as you know, first I thought about Mr. Ribotton, my former science teacher. Mr. Ribotton and his rules for experiments. His son was in my class, his name was Maxime. Maxime Ribotton: a shifty, clammy kid whose dream in life was to become a police inspector. I have no idea what's become of him, but I have no idea what's become of most of my classmates at the Lycée Jan-son de Sailly. We lost contact. I blame myself for not doing more to stay in touch with these old friends, even the ones I was closest to. Emmanuel Guilhen, for instance, my best friend in eighth and ninth grade. Both of us liked to read the satirical weekly *Charlie Hebdo*, whose spirit of derision we loved and copied. Since he lived just two blocks away, we met up and walked to school together. From Rue Ray-nouard, where I lived, I walked up Rue Vineuse, at the end of which I met Emmanuel Guilhen, who'd come down from Rue Benjamin Franklin. From there it was straight ahead, Rue Scheffer, Rue Scheffer, Rue Scheffer, crossing Avenue Paul Doumer, Rue Louis David, Rue Cortambert—quiet, opulent streets in Paris's Sixteenth Arrondissement— before reaching Avenue Georges Mandel with its beautiful chestnut trees, which we just needed to cross to enter the lycée through the gate on Rue Decamps. How many times did I walk this route? Twice a day, five days a week, thirty or so weeks a year for six years . . . I can see it perfectly. It took all of twenty minutes, and I could spend twenty minutes going over it in my mind. I can also see perfectly the apartment where I grew up. My parents haven't lived there for a long time. I'll have to go see them when I get back. I don't see them often enough. I should take my fa-ther to lunch at the restaurant on Quai des Grands Au-gustins, like I used to do every month. Will I tell him what I've been doing for the past ten days? Ten days of sitting in silence on a cushion, focusing on my nostrils? Would it amuse him? Would it interest him if I could make him see everything that's at stake in this seemingly grotesque

practice? Would it worry him? Would he think I've joined a
cult? That's certainly what my mother would think, unless
I told her I was doing it for a book. If it's for a book, okay,
she's always game. A book justifies anything. When my sisters and I were little, she told us that it didn't matter if we
got bad grades at school so long as we read books. Even if
he complains that it's getting worse with age, my father has
an amazing memory. To get to sleep, he can visualize in
the minutest detail an apartment where we lived fifty years
ago—room by room, wall by wall, painting by painting,
right down to the contents of each drawer. Sometimes before going to sleep I do something similar, remembering as
precisely as possible the day that's just passed. When you
do this exercise you shouldn't go too fast or skim over too
many details, otherwise you'll be done in two minutes. For
example: got up, yoga, breakfast with the family, Patanjali at the Café de l'Église, work, lunch with Olivier, more
work, dinner with the family, two episodes of *In Treatment*,
and now bed, where I'm going over my day. There, done,
only a little too fast. That said, you shouldn't go too slow
or go into too much detail either, because if you start list-
ing everything involved in preparing breakfast, for example, it can go on forever. It's hardly an exaggeration to say
that a whole day, and maybe even a whole life, wouldn't
be enough to *fully* describe that quarter of an hour spent
making breakfast. As usual you have to find the right balance. An account that gives sufficient detail but lasts no
longer than, say, fifteen or twenty minutes. For me, twenty
minutes is the length of an average meditation session. It's
a good length, a natural length, like ninety minutes for a

film. I wonder if something like going over your day can be considered a form of meditation, or if it's not the very opposite: something far too hands-on, too obsessive? Twenty minutes is also the average amount of time you need to do the form of tai chi. Will I talk about tai chi in my book? Yes, of course. Memories of tai chi clearly belong in a book on yoga. I use the word *yoga* very broadly: tai chi is a form of yoga. Sex can be a form of yoga. Will I talk about the woman who gave me the Gemini statue? Or the light at the Hotel Cornavin? What is certain is that I'll say more about the Bardo, and in that context about a fantastic short story I read as an adolescent. It impressed me enormously, and I still remember it—vividly if confusedly—as being inspired by the Bardo in a way that's as powerful as Philip K. Dick's *Ubik*. It's by George Langelaan, who's (quite) well known for having written "The Fly," of which two excellent screen versions have been made. Cronenberg's, of course, but also the first one, a B movie with Vincent Price. I think about all the sci-fi and horror stories I've read since my teens, all of which remain clear in my mind. I haven't forgotten a single one. Why do I like them so much? Why do they mean so much to me? Why do such stories help me understand my own? I passed this taste on to my two sons, and sometimes I can't help worrying why, like me, they're so susceptible to it. Can meditation tame the sense of horror that lurks under the surface of my life? Does it have access to all of human experience, or are there doors it can't go through? What can it do for people whose bodies or minds have failed them? One can't help wondering: If you were plunged into such an abyss—multiple sclerosis, schizophrenia, locked-in syndrome, extreme mental distress—could you tame your desperate situation with meditation? Could you learn to inhabit this uninhabitable self? There are examples: Stephen Hawking, from what I gather, said that meditation allowed him to live within the prison of his paralyzed body. If it were me, I think I'd collapse and want to kill myself. I wonder what meditation could be like for a schizophrenic. What would it be like to take a calm look inside yourself, when inside yourself is threatening enemy territory, the site of untold, interminable, boundless horror? Horror that never stops, and that takes up all the space, 100 percent of the mental pie, of which we devote just 20 percent to the present, according to Chögyam Trungpa. Where did Chögyam Trungpa get that figure? It's obviously absurd, yet it interests me. Anything that helps me get a better understanding of mental activity interests me. I've always been interested in my own mental activity, to the point of making it my trade. A long time ago, when I was just starting out as an author, I came across a piece of advice to apprentice writers, which I love, quoted by Freud. He cites a certain Ludwig Börne, who was a minor figure of German Romanticism. Like Glenn Gould's maxim about the state of wonder and serenity, these words have been a sort of mantra that has accompanied me for much of my life:

> Take a few sheets of paper and for three days on end write down, without fabrication or hypocrisy, everything that comes into your head. Write down what you think of yourself, of your wife, of the Turkish War, of Goethe, of Fonk's trial, of the Last Judgment,

of your superiors—and when three days have passed you will be quite out of your senses with astonishment at the new and unheard-of thoughts you have had. This is the art of becoming an original writer in three days.

Becoming an original writer—whether in three days or three years or thirty years—was the obsession of my youth, and it's been with me ever since. I've often wondered who Fonk was, what crime he committed (even Wikipedia draws a blank), and if Ludwig Börne has bequeathed anything to literature aside from this memorable advice (no). The writers who write what goes through their heads are the ones I prefer. Montaigne, our patron saint, does just that. He writes what occurs to him, regally indifferent to those who say they don't care about what occurs to him and that one would have to be very pretentious, very egocentric, to keep a record of such things. Because he himself believes that there's nothing more interesting, and that it's all the more interesting in that he's an ordinary man. Not one whose memoirs are read because of all the brilliant things he's done, but one whose only quality is to be a man, and who for this reason can testify to what it is to be a man without being encumbered by any exceptional status whatsoever.

'Tis a rugged road, more so than it seems, to follow a pace so rambling and uncertain, as that of the soul; to penetrate the dark profundities of its intricate internal windings; to choose and lay hold of so many little nimble motions. 'Tis now many years since that

> my thoughts have had no other aim and level than
> myself, and that I have only pried into and studied
> myself: or, if I study any other thing, 'tis to apply it
> to or rather in myself. There is no description so dif-
> ficult, nor doubtless of so great utility, as that of a
> man's self . . .

That said, as far as difficulty goes, when Ludwig Börne
recommends that we write what goes through our heads
"without fabrication or hypocrisy," in my opinion he takes
things a bit far. "Without hypocrisy" is okay: I think it's
entirely possible to write in an unhypocritical way, and I
believe I do just that. But "without fabrication"! Börne slips
this in as if it were no more than a technical detail, whereas
in fact it's the crux, the unattainable goal of the whole en-
terprise. Writing down everything that goes through your
head "without fabrication" is exactly the same as observing
your breathing without modifying it. Which is to say: it's
impossible. Still, it's worth trying. It's worth spending your
whole life trying. That's what I do, it's my karma, I can't do
anything else but use words to make sentences, sentences
to make paragraphs, paragraphs to fill pages, pages to make
chapters, and—if I'm lucky—chapters to make books. I
think about it all the time. The two biggest parts of my
mental pie are dedicated to thoughts about work and fantasies about sex. Sexual fantasies occupy between a quarter
and a third of the pie, I'd say, most often at certain privileged moments: before I fall asleep, when I can't sleep at
all, all the border zones between waking and slumber.
Only, what turns me on about these fantasies is simply

their being *possible*—and not very fanciful at all. On the contrary, they're realistic, even painstakingly so. The faces and bodies I summon to satisfy them must be those of women with whom it would be possible for me to actually sleep, today, without it being either overly improbable or a complete transgression. For example, I've never jerked off thinking about a woman I don't know and stand little chance of getting to know, like a famous actress or model. But there is a scenario I come back to again and again. I think it must be inspired by a film I once saw, Jarmusch's *Broken Flowers*, with Bill Murray. In the film Murray gets a letter telling him he has a son, and he goes on a tour of his past lovers—and sleeps with more than one, as I recall—to get to the bottom of things. There must be four or five of them, and that's about the number of women I'd go see given the chance: the peaks of my erotic life. I love this story, and I love imagining in detail and almost in real time the night I'd spend with each. What we'd say, how we'd make love. I remember how I made love with every single one, it's the stuff of endless reveries. Desiring someone who desires me and losing interest quickly enough in someone who loses interest in me has been a constant in my love life that, even if I've known other pangs—God knows—has at least spared me the ordeals of men who go on loving women who despise them, ignore them, or lead them along. Of course, I have desired women who weren't interested in me: I tried my luck and if it didn't work, I got over it. Because since they weren't attracted to me, I quickly stopped being attracted to them. Sure, I've had unhappy love affairs, but no one-sided passions. No eroticism without reciprocity, understanding, and realism. Love is complicated for me, as I guess it is for everyone. Not sex, though, which is no doubt the human relationship I'm most comfortable with, and which shows me in my best light. I don't attach any guilt to it, it's a refuge, not an abyss, it doesn't corrupt my soul. I wouldn't say the same about my thoughts about work, which come in two very different categories depending on whether I'm working on a project or not. If I am, if I have a book in progress and if I've reached cruising speed in writing it, then I only think about that, I write sentence after sentence after sentence, there's no time for anything else. Along with sex (sometimes), these are the paramount moments of my life, when I think it's worth it to be on earth. When I'm not working, on the other hand, thoughts about work tend to be of the wrong sort, namely anticipations of success, glory, and importance. These, then, make me feel guilty and even humiliate me. Visualizing a night of lovemaking in every detail I find not only pleasant but also good and healthy. Imagining what people—which people?—will say about me, which glowing rumors will waft my way, makes me ashamed. Unfortunately, it's just part of my mental wiring. Right now, sitting on my zafu in the Morvan region, a good half of my thoughts are about this book on yoga, which is to be called *Exhaling*, and I'm perhaps more caught up with it than I realize, since I'm thinking very much about the book itself and not about how successful it'll be or what people will say about it. I draw up the plan, go over and over my list of definitions of meditation. I wonder what I'll say about Vipassana. I try to imagine how it might be to transcribe with as little fabrication as possible everything that goes through my head during this two-hour session: basically what you're reading here, only I'd have to add everything that's taking place at the same time with my breathing and sensations. The moments when I let myself be carried far from them by the vritti, the moments when I realize I've let myself be carried away and I return to them again. The moments when the vritti take control, and the rarer times when, because I'm observing them, I have a little control over them. That said, these vritti aren't all that bad. What I've just transcribed could be called letting your mind wander, or even—to be indulgent—thinking. There's a sentence by Schopenhauer that makes me laugh a lot: "The best way to think smart things is not to think twaddle." In fact, what makes me laugh in this sentence isn't Schopenhauer but his French translator and his use of the word *fadaises*, or twaddle. "Thinking twaddle": an idea that fleetingly crossed my mind a few lines back keeps pestering me. Is that what these thoughts that have been coming thick and fast as I've been sitting here are? Twaddle? I mean, sure, they're not great. Nevertheless they're good, respectable, human thoughts: varied enough, and interesting enough. Suddenly I can't help wondering why Patanjali and his clan view these harmless vritti as if they were swarms of harmful insects, enemies that must be quashed at all costs and replaced by observations of air passing through nostrils. Suddenly I have a doubt. What am I doing here? What did I get caught up in? Why should I be ashamed to think what I think? Isn't this a bit like North Korea, after all? Rest assured, I'm not comparing myself with Montaigne. But wouldn't Patanjali also condemn Montaigne for his complacency regarding his vritti? For the sheer pleasure he takes in following "a pace so rambling and uncertain as that of the soul," in choosing and laying hold of "so many little nimble motions"? That said, though, when push comes to shove my favorite sentence is still Captain Haddock's memorable line, the one I thought about a while ago, and which I think about quite often, in fact: "It's both very simple and very complicated." Are there things in life that aren't both very simple and very complicated? Things that are only simple, or only complicated? Which of the Tintin books does he say it in? *Land of Black Gold*? *The Calculus Affair*? The first time I made love with the woman who would give me the Gemini statue, it was at the Hotel Cornavin in Geneva, where a scene—also memorable—from *The Calculus Affair* takes place. We'd both just been at a yoga retreat in Morges, a small town on the shores of Lake Geneva. I watched her often during the sessions, and she told me later that she'd noticed. On the last day, most of us took the train to Geneva, from where I had to go back to Paris and she to I don't know where. But that's not what happened. What happened—which I had absolutely not foreseen but she had, she told me later— was that after exchanging glances, without a word being said, we left the Gare de Genève-Cornavin together, walked over to the Hotel Cornavin, which is just across the road, took one of the elevators drawn so exactly by Hergé in *The Calculus Affair*, and a few minutes later were lying together on a large bed, which turned out to be made up of two small beds that split apart as soon as we started to move. We made love for a very long time that afternoon, although all in all we didn't move that much. I was a premature ejaculator in my youth, and that has given me a taste for slowness. The women I've got along best with sexually share the same taste. Postponing, delaying, prolonging. Staying on the cusp. Oddly enough, at first we lay together like spoons for a long time, me behind her. I say oddly enough, because it's unusual for two people who've just met and are dying to have sex to start by lying together for a long moment, peacefully and unhurriedly, in this position of shared confidence that is more conducive to falling asleep. At one point I let out a deep sigh of total well-being, the way you let all your tension go, and said, "I feel good," and she whispered, "Me too." She reached behind her, took my right hand and placed it on her right breast, and we stayed like that for some time. My hand cupping her breast, we were totally receptive to all the sensations in my palm and the tip of her breast, which stiffened, and stiffened all the more as I wasn't kneading or squeezing it. On the contrary, I withdrew my hand slightly—without moving it, that is—so that instead her breast pushed against my palm, and I felt the skin of her nipple as it grew taut and erect. I became erect too, but coolly, calmly, pressing as much of my skin against hers as possible. Inch by inch, we increased this area. By relaxing a muscle, then contracting it, then relaxing it again, we gained a little surface contact, it was minute but steady, really it was a form of yoga. You could say we started making love by doing yoga, and that we continued doing yoga by making love. A little later I was inside her, with deep, slow thrusts. I pulled out farther and farther, almost coming out of her, she pushed her pelvis toward mine so as not to lose me, I was hanging on the edge, we both made the moment last, and then I sank back into her, slower and slower, deeper and deeper, just like in meditation when your breathing becomes slower and deeper, the inhalation grows longer, the exhalation grows longer, as does the pause between the two when you're sure the movement is at the end of its cycle and will start again in the other direction. But instead it continues, intensifies, deepens, with all your sensations homing in on that point. We must have stayed like that for an hour, maybe two, without changing our position—I almost wrote: our posture. Each gesture increased our pleasure and our astonishment. In the end I was resting on her entirely, with no part of my body touching the bed—my legs on hers, my toes propped against her insteps, my arms wrapped around her shoulders, my hands caressing her face. We moved very slowly, as if we were at the bottom of the sea, I only shifted the weight that bore down on her, thrusting very deep, lightening up a little, with tiny variations in the contact between our hips and torsos, she accompanying my withdrawals, welcoming my thrusts. Little by little, we stopped moving. We weren't moving at all, my sex wasn't moving at all, it was only hers that contracted slowly, regularly, around mine, like a breath. Our faces were very close, we'd stop kissing only to look into each other's eyes, each knowing that we were feeling exactly what the other was. Though we hadn't spoken to each other yet that morning and didn't even know each other's last name, I felt like I was her, I told her, she felt like she was me, and it was at this moment, when we were so together, when we did no more than press as tightly as possible against each other, each commingled with and almost inside the other, that she asked me if I saw the light, and I saw it then, the light above her, the light above us, it seems silly to say it like that, but this light, which was at the same time infinitely distant and a halo that enveloped us, was like what people who've lived through a near-death experience describe, it's as impossible to describe as it is to reproduce, but when you experience it, you're certain that it's not an illusion or autosuggestion, that it's the real thing. We repeated to ourselves in amazement: *it's real*.

The path

The center is located in an old farmhouse, in the middle of a forest. Between each two-hour meditation session you can walk in the woods, without straying from a path that's fenced off on both sides. So we pass one another in silence on this path bordered by bare trees, carpeted with dead leaves, and dotted with large, muddy puddles, the way monks must pass one another in a monastery. Everyone keeps their eyes to the ground, their hoods pulled over their foreheads like cowls. While I avoid meeting my companions' gaze, that doesn't stop me from observing them. They're lost in thought, and I wonder what they could be thinking. I observe their gait, I observe my own. The path takes you around in a circle, which you can cover in about ten minutes. Depending on how fast you walk, of course. Ten minutes for the average stride, three to four miles per hour. We were asked last night not to run, so as

not to disrupt the others' concentration. Walking slowly—
and even walking very slowly—isn't forbidden, however. So
I slowly place the heel of one foot on the uneven, slippery
ground. It would be better to do this barefoot on a parquet floor, but I have good shoes with soles that are flexible
enough to allow me to roll my foot—or imagine that I'm
rolling it—from the heel to the sole, then to the ball, and
then finally to the tips of my five toes, trying all the while
to feel each one clearly. As I do so, I keep my weight on my
back leg with the foot sunk into the earth, rooted as firmly
as possible. Then, slowly, very slowly, I transfer my weight
to my front leg. I try to do this the way you'd pour a heavy,
sticky liquid like honey from one vessel into another: not
drop by drop, but in a continuous flow. I fill my front foot
by slowing it down, and empty my back foot by keeping my
weight on it as if I were reluctant to move on. And between
the two I make the movement last as long as possible, alert
to each step of the process. The banal movement of walking, which comes down to putting one foot in front of the
other, I try to do in full awareness, breaking it down, slowing it and observing each passing sensation, the contact
with the soil, with the air, the temperature. As it turns out,
I'm not the only one here practicing this sort of meditation
in movement: the guy in front of me is standing on one leg
like a heron, and I identify him as a practitioner of tai chi
as clearly as I identified the guy who grabbed his ass earlier as a practitioner of Iyengar yoga. And seeing me walk
in slow motion, he too will no doubt be able to situate me
as well. This silent, secret complicity is one of the things I
loved at the dojo.

The longest distance between two points

There was a joke at the Dojo de la Montagne that could also be a Zen koan: Everyone knows that the shortest distance between two points is a straight line. But the longest? Everyone also knows that certain people can run fast, that some can run faster than others, and that at every moment in history there is one human being who can run faster than all the rest. At the time I'm writing the record was— and still is—held by a Jamaican athlete called Usain Bolt. I don't know who it'll be when you read this, no doubt someone else because these records that seem unbeatable are made to be broken. In any case, a speed record is easy to measure. But a slowness record?

The form

Wall to wall, the dojo was roughly twenty yards in length. One time it took me an hour to cross it. The next day I tried to beat my record and go even slower. The hard part about this exercise isn't so much walking slowly as it is doing it *without a break*. Without any jolts or jerks, without breaking stride. In a continuous, fluid, uninterrupted movement. It's like swimming in space, and it's a hugely effective way of focusing your attention. In the long process of learning tai chi, it's also a preparatory exercise for the study of what's called "the form," a sequence of movements that, executed at an average speed, takes about twenty minutes to accomplish. There are several variations of the form, each one associated with a very old Chinese school, the two best-known being the Chen style and the Yang style. At the Dojo de la Montagne we preferred the Yang style. First you work on the movements one by one, then little by little you put them together, the way a pianist works on a sonata. They say three hours are enough to learn the rules of the board game go, but that it takes three lives to master it. It also takes at least three lives to master tai chi, but rather than three hours it takes more like three years merely to memorize the series of movements that serve as a framework for the practice itself, and to begin to understand *what they're for*. You cannot be in a hurry. You have to consent, for months on end, to do nothing more than walk in slow motion on the parquet floors of the dojo. Then a moment comes when you start doing what you did when you were walking with the more complicated movements that make up the form, which have pretty Chinese names like grasping the bird's tail, playing the lute, repulsing the monkey, cloud hands . . .

Tai chi in the metro

Anyone who practices a martial art will understand sooner or later that it's not about successfully performing the movements but about making something happen inside you. About curtailing your ego, your greed, your thirst for competition and conquest, about educating your conscience to allow it unfiltered access to reality, to things as they are. Anything you apply yourself to with love and dedication, from kung fu to motorcycle maintenance, can be called yoga. It's in this spirit that I once practiced tai chi—in this spirit and, I repeat to put my wisdom in perspective, completely plastered two nights out of three. I loved feeling the movements of the form as they became engraved in my memory. I loved it when one gesture followed another without my having to think about it, as if on its own, as naturally as breathing. I dreamed of writing like that: with the sort of fluidity, ease, and calm that were—and are—more accessible to me when I do tai chi or yoga—since I'll always be an amateur on that front—than on my own terrain, where the inextricable knot of obsession, megalomania, and the noble desire to do a good job that constitutes a writer's ego reigns supreme. With as much care as I take in writing, rereading, and rewriting sentences, I performed and repeated the same gestures over and over again, each new attempt building on the memory of the previous ones, while gaining in precision and finesse. Every chance I had, I practiced the form. Taking the metro became a pleasure. I stood near the pole in the center of the car but didn't hold on to it, and, letting my arms hang at my side, I practiced keeping my balance. The metro's moving, however, jolting and joggling in an irregular and unpredictable way as it turns, speeds up, slows down, and slams on the brakes. Although you can't anticipate these shocks, you can try to move with them and absorb them in your feet, ankles, calves, thighs, and hips. Being careful not to attract attention or flail your arms, you twist and bend like a flame. It's rare that you don't lose your balance and grab on to the bar at least once between stations. But it can also happen that you absorb a jerk that should have thrown you off, or that you totter and catch yourself, losing and recovering your balance. And no one around you can see that you're riding the train like a bucking bronco. It's a thrill.

Cloud hands

In my group of beginners there was a small woman in her fifties. She was a little chubby and very nice, and she'd taken up tai chi a year earlier without expecting much or even suspecting that it could be anything but a healthy, not too strenuous form of exercise. One morning, she came to class with her eyes shining, overwhelmed, panting but happy: she looked like she'd just made love. She'd come by metro as usual, and in a long, deserted corridor two young guys had attacked her and tried to steal her purse. "And then something happened, I didn't really understand what. I did cloud hands, and the guy who'd grabbed my arm hit the wall with his head, and the two ran off without looking back." When we heard this, our eyes started to shine as well, and we all probably looked like we'd just made love too. It's something everyone who practices a martial art wonders: Would the combat techniques I'm learning help me in a real street fight? Faced with edgy, violent attackers who are not afraid to inflict pain? The small woman's exploit was an answer to this question, and an encouraging one at that. Under Pascal's particularly enthusiastic guidance, that morning we performed cloud hands again and again—this apparently peaceful, meditative movement that had so conveniently forged a path in the neurons of the small woman, who that day became our real-life heroine. Unlike on other days, we all stayed and talked after class. Yes, Pascal told us, tai chi really is a martial art. Each movement of the form is an attack or a parry. People tend to think of it as a gentle sort of gymnastics that elderly Chinese people do in parks, but as a means of self-defense it's every bit as dangerous as karate or Thai boxing, something that more advanced students know all too well. I knew that there were courses for more advanced students at the Dojo de la Montagne, but I couldn't see myself taking them for another couple of years at least. "Think again," Pascal said. "You can come. Watch what others do and copy it. That's how you improve." In this way I came to join the advanced group and started attending Dr. Yang's annual seminar.

Fast and slow

The seminar lasted a week, six hours a day. During that time, I was in a world of my own. Many practitioners came from all over France, Germany, Spain, and Italy. They brought sleeping bags and slept in the dojo, which smelled a bit like feet. Dr. Yang was an easygoing, cheerful man in his fifties, of average build and looks. He didn't go on and on about spirituality or play the guru, and he took pride in the fact that his school also turned a profit. He watched what we were doing, corrected us with a gesture, and rarely demonstrated, but his demonstrations were dazzling. One day he showed us a sequence of the form:

three or four movements that took me about a minute when I did them as slowly as I could. He did them in twenty-five. And during those twenty-five minutes he must have breathed twice: two inhalations and two exhalations, his breath circulating with limitless scope and slowness in his body, which moved like a jellyfish or sea anemone. I've never seen anyone do something so impressive. Gathered in a circle around Dr. Yang, we didn't dare so much as breathe for fear of interrupting this miraculous flow. And then, when he got to the end of a movement that was so prolonged that it looked like he wasn't moving at all, it was like a snake darting out its tongue. In a flash, the front of his body uncoiled at the speed of light, the index and middle finger of his right hand spread to sink into the eyes of a virtual opponent, and he looked at us, laughed his little laugh, and barked: "Don't miss the point, it's to kill!" We were all transfixed, but Dr. Yang didn't give us time to recover. He squinted, still laughing, and said, "Now, fast," and disappeared. I'm not kidding, I'm not exaggerating. It was as if he'd entered another dimension and was moving so fast that we could only catch a glimpse of his wake. He'd been there, he was gone. He now did this sequence that we'd been doing in a minute and that he'd just stretched out over twenty-five in a few seconds, too fast for the eye to follow his movements, and yet we could be sure that nothing was rushed, nothing had been omitted, and everything was there, right down to the tiniest nuances. Imagine a scene in a movie that's shown first in slow motion, slowed down twenty-four times, say, then in fast motion, twenty-four times the normal speed. That's what Dr. Yang did right there in front of us. First Master Yoda, then Bruce Lee. With astonishing authority, he showed us that day that tai chi was as much the one as the other, and that we shouldn't just do the form at our customary, plodding *andante ma non troppo* tempo, but also as slowly and as fast as we could: to meditate, and to kill.

At the same time

And that wasn't all. Dr. Yang still had another card up his sleeve. No spectacular demonstration this time, just a few words that he tossed our way on the last day of the seminar with one of his little laughs. "If you've understood that you need to practice the form not just slowly but also quickly, that's good. Now you must understand that it's not enough to work slowly and quickly: you have to do both *at the same time*."

"Advance your feet backward!"

The expression "at the same time" has been compromised in France, because of its use and overuse by our current president, Emmanuel Macron, to the point that just saying it is already a joke. Nevertheless I understand what lies behind it, perhaps only too well. Whenever I think something, I tend to immediately think the opposite as well. In fact I'm so quick to see other people's point of view that I often agree with the last person who spoke. In the sense that Dr. Yang used it, though, the expression was anything but a joke. And it's the key not only to tai chi, but to all varieties of yoga. One of my teachers is Toni d'Amelio. She's American, and she loves popular French expressions. She puts things another way. When you do yoga, she says, you have to want *"le beurre et l'argent du beurre."* This phrase is often used to denigrate the profiteer, someone who seeks to exploit a situation and reap all the benefits while avoiding the disadvantages. But when Toni applies it to yoga, it takes on a different meaning. It's about cultivating—by stretching, doing the postures, and uniting the body and the mind under the yoke of the asanas—qualities we believe are contradictory and between which we feel we have to choose: flexibility and strength, slowness and speed, stillness and movement, meditation and action. In fact you don't have to choose. You don't have to sacrifice one thing for another. Any given posture is made up of endless movements, and the most sweeping movements emanate from a core of stillness. In going downward you must go up, in going upward you must go down, when you push you must pull, when you pull you must push, you must play the midfield and the attack, want one thing and its opposite, have your cake and eat it, never mind what the English say. And I still remember how we all laughed in delight when Toni ordered: "Advance your feet backward!"

The voice of the French interpreter

It's dinnertime, but there's no dinner: Buddhist monks'
fare. Instead, after the last meditation of the day, we listen
to a speech by S. N. Goenka. We're no longer in posture
and can sit as we want. So long as we don't turn our feet
toward the altar, we can even lie sprawled on our cushions.
I'm tired but happy. The first day went well. No posture
problems, my breathing was calm, my thoughts didn't stray
too far, and my tai chi memories came back: I've often
thought that all that work wasn't lost, that the form was
stored somewhere in the depths of my mind and would re-
surface one day. Regardless of what people say on the forums about cramming and brainwashing, Vipassana makes
a good impression on me. And one thing that makes a particularly good impression is the voice of the interpreter who
translates the speeches recorded in Pali by S. N. Goenka

into French, two or three minutes at a time. S. N. Goenka's voice is the voice of an old man. In it you can hear his age, the Ganges, the nearness of death, and something much, much older than S. N. Goenka himself. The voice of his interpreter belongs to a young man: clear, distinct, calm—more the voice of an affable, educated young man than that of a sage. It's not the voice of a guru, it has none of the pervasive, obscene warmth of the professionals of persuasion—politicians, preachers, and performers who are sure of their charm—and I wasn't at all surprised to learn afterward that it belongs to a baroque singer and Vipassana follower who practices karma yoga by putting his talent in the service of the master. Listening to him, I think of what Roland Barthes, so sensitive to what he called the "grain" of the voice, praised in his favorite per-formers: fully intelligible diction, which sacrifices nothing but at the same time doesn't make a big thing out of every syllable; natural phrasing, without affectation but without overdoing the absence of affectation, an ideal balance be-tween distance and familiarity. And the liaisons between syllables. Ah, the liaisons! They're *the* touchstone in the art of saying a text in French. And a real brain-teaser. Must they *all* be pronounced? Not all of them, no. Because come on: some of them are just a pain and should be avoided. But where do you draw the line, then, between overdo-ing your diction—which quickly becomes pedantic—and talking too casually, which, if done systematically, also sounds affected? Listening attentively to S. N. Goenka's interpreter, I'm stunned. Because there's no getting around it: he pronounces *all* the liaisons. Yet you'd never notice it. It's as if he didn't, yet he does: it's great art, vocal yoga, and I say to myself that this guy demonstrates the same virtues of accuracy, simplicity, and naturalness in giving expression to his old master's words that I look for when I write. As the *I Ching*, the ancient book of divination that is at the source and heart of Chinese thought, says: "Perfect grace consists not in exterior ornamentation of the substance, but in the simple fitness of its form."

The evening speech

"We are miserable," says S. N. Goenka. "Very miserable.

"We are subject to suffering.

"The fact that we exist in space and time, whether we're humans, flies, or gods, condemns us to this suffering that, together with perpetual change, is the law of existence.

"Suffering, perpetual change, fear, greed, aversion.

"Misery.

"The cause of this misery is ignorance.

"Ignorance is confusing our mind with what we call 'me.' It's the identification with this 'me' that creates misery.

"So you must ask yourself: What is it in you that says 'Me! Me! Me!'?

"You must investigate.

"There's no point doing it intellectually. There's no point reading books on Buddhism. That's like reading a menu over and over instead of eating.

"You must investigate yourself.

"You must look inside yourself to see what is saying 'Me! Me! Me!'

"You must delve into the depths of yourself. It's in crossing these depths that you'll reach reality.

"The only tool you have to reach reality, the only raft you have to make the crossing, is your body.

"Apart from a scanty knowledge of anatomy, you don't know anything about your body.

"You're here to explore it.

"You're here to explore it through your sensations and your breathing. Above all your breathing.

"Today you started to observe your breathing.

"You'll continue tomorrow. And in the days to come.

"You'll work hard. With persistence, patience, and calm.

"You're not going to reach liberation in ten days, but you will acquire a technique that can help to take you there.

"It's a very safe technique, it's been around for a very long time, many people have reached liberation thanks to it.

"This is a technique, not a religion. It doesn't work with ideas or beliefs, but with the breath. And the breath is something real.

"Don't work with ideas or beliefs, only with your breath. Only with your direct experience.

"You're not being asked to believe anything. Absolutely not.

"Don't believe: try. Take the plunge.

"The first day is over, there are nine left.

"In general, the second and sixth days are the hardest.

"That might not be your case, but it's good to be prepared.

"You've come here to operate on your mind.

"This is good for you, but it can be painful. It can even be dangerous.

"Strange and disturbing things can surface.

"You might be afraid, you might cry.

"You might get fed up with not having dinner.

"Persevere. Hold out until the tenth day. After that you can say it was silly, or not for you. But only then.

"Now go and sleep."

I fidget

For me the second day starts with a complete disaster. I've known people who counted their hours of meditation the way airline employees count their flight hours. How many meditation hours have I chalked up? Am I entitled to miles? I started twenty-five years ago. If I'd practiced all that time for half an hour a day, I could multiply 25 by 365 and then divide by 2: close to five thousand hours. That would be nice. Five thousand hours of meditation, or of driving, or of sex, or of any activity is hard to describe. In any case, though, I'm far, far off the mark. I practiced so irregularly, so erratically, with such long breaks in between . . . That said, I'm not a beginner either. I have no problem doing the lotus, starting with the right foot or with the left, and on the strength of that I said to myself: okay, the vritti will no doubt take some work, but at least my posture should be fine. Not by a long shot. Today things just don't work. Very quickly my back starts to hurt, I get a sharp pain in the middle of my right shoulder. Sharp, but not piercing: it's nothing unbearable, I should be able to get rid of it with a little concentration. Is the pain in the middle of my shoulder as I first thought, or underneath it? More like underneath it. I can't really imagine the muscles under my shoulder blade, what they're attached to and how, but I try to go at the problem with the "have your cake and eat it too" technique, exerting pressure both from the outside in and from the inside out, in the hope of isolating my shoulder blade and with it the pain. I focus on my shoulder, not on the pain. Despite my resolve to observe and not to act, and above all to sit still no matter what, I'm now discreetly—very discreetly—rotating my shoulder. No doubt the movement's invisible, but I know I've screwed up. The first defeat is a stepping-stone to all further defeats: already I'm starting over. I roll my shoulder, and roll it again. I twist and fidget. And now—while I'm at it—far too early I let myself do the long, undulating movement usually reserved for the end of the session, letting my head fall forward, pulled down by its own weight. A head's a heavy thing: easily ten pounds or more. My neck sags, my chin presses against my collarbone, my chest hollows, my back becomes rounded. It's what's called the back arch, or cat pose. With the help of exhalation and gravity, you let your head drop down as far as possible, as if you wanted to touch your belly button with the tip of your nose. You give in, surrender. Then when you reach your limit you stay that way, as low as possible, bending as far forward as you can, and, when you're sure you can't descend any more, very slowly, inhaling this time, you start to raise your head, your forehead, as if a thread were pulling you by the nose, but this time forward and upward. And with this upward movement everything that was folded unfolds, everything that was sagging straightens out, what was concave becomes convex, the back unbends in a slow and continuous movement, you return to the initial posture, and how good that feels. This movement, comprising two successive movements, one subsiding and the other rising, one renouncing and the other vanquishing, one exhaling and the other inhaling, is wonderfully pleasant, and what's more it's massaged my shoulder, the pain has receded. The only problem is that I've shot my load far too early. I feel better sitting in posture now, but as with all compulsions—cigarettes, alcohol, cocaine—you shouldn't start because after a short moment of satisfaction all you want is to start all over again. I resolve to take ten deep, very slow breaths before allowing my head to drop again, but in fact I take only five or six and down I plunge, slumping forward once again. I bend as far as possible, sinking as far and as long as I can before rising once more, coming back to the posture I now suspect I'll hold for even less time than the last. I can't stop fidgeting, slouching and straightening, and, now that I've come this far, I open my eyes. Is everyone twisting and turning like me?

There are no grown-ups

In front of me is a wall of erect, compact backs, motionless under the blue, conical blankets that fall around them

like tepees. What's going on underneath? What's going on
in their bodies? In their minds? I look at the backs, I look
at the necks. I wonder who's in pain like me, who's bored,
who's daydreaming, who's freaking out. There are a lot of
freaked-out people in places like this. In fact there are a
lot just about everywhere, but perhaps even more among
the seekers of meaning and serenity. It's a funny, touching
sight, one hundred and twenty people gathered for ten days
in a huge hall to delve into themselves and get a better
handle on who they are and what moves them. Each of us
is caught up with their own thoughts and obsessions, each
is trapped in their own turmoil, each runs up against their
own dead ends. Each of us came here hoping to see a little
more clearly, to extricate themself from their own particular mess—if only just a bit—and to be a little less unhappy.
The writer André Malraux relates a discussion he had with
an old priest: "You've spent fifty years listening to people
in the secrecy of the confessional, what have you learned
about the human soul?" The priest: "Two things. First of
all, people are much more unhappy than one thinks. And
second, there is no such thing as grown-ups." There are no
grown-ups: under our clothes we're all naked. Whomever
we meet, we're always right to imagine them naked under
their clothes, their pale, fragile, insecure bodies, and the
scared little boy or lost little girl they were before they became the president of France or the famous actress they
now are. That goes for Emmanuel Macron and Catherine
Deneuve as much as it does for Mr. Ribotton. Forty-five
years on, I can't quite separate in my mind my eighth-grade
teacher Mr. Ribotton from his reincarnation just a few feet

to my right. What's on the mind of this reborn Ribotton?
What's he fighting? Where are his vritti taking him? Is he
still developing his rules for experiments, over and over
again, with every noisy breath he takes? Can his smug insights patch the immense sorrow inside him? What is it
like to be Mr. Ribotton? Perhaps that's the most interesting
thing in life, trying to figure out what it's like to be someone
else. That's one of the reasons people write books, another
being to discover what it's like to be yourself. I mostly think
about the latter. Probably too much. Recently it struck me
that my friend Hélène F. starts most of her sentences with
"You," while I start most of mine with "I." That got me
thinking. According to a somewhat passé rule of etiquette,
you shouldn't start a letter with "I." That's a rule I'd do well
to follow, in my life as well as in my work. Not an easy task.
Beyond reach? It's a big topic. Simone Weil—again—said
there are few people, ultimately, who know that others exist. Who, quite simply, are *aware* of that: that others exist.
Meditation—eleventh definition—should make you aware
of just that. If it doesn't, if it remains something you share
only with yourself, it's useless: just another narcissistic
plaything. Suddenly I'm afraid that, at least for me, that's
what it is, just another narcissistic plaything. That makes
me sad.

Hugging trees

As I walk sadly in the woods, some people are watching the trees. Some squat in front of a stump and observe it pensively. Some stroke a trunk, feel its bark, open to all the sensations caused by the contact of the wood on their skin. Others stare at a broad oak tree, then give it a big hug. Their arms surround it, their hands caress it, their faces rub against its bark, eyes half closed in ecstasy. It's a familiar New Age practice, hugging and stroking trees to commune with Gaia, the spirit of the earth, and I wonder if it would have occurred to those who do it if they hadn't been told it was the done thing, that it's a sign of sensitivity, connection with nature, letting go and whatnot. I flee my sadness with irony. It's a classic ruse to which I've resorted many times. I latch on to a negative thought, one I should really keep at arm's length, and it leads me to another, even more negative one that's all the more efficient because it's terribly convincing. A few days before I left for the retreat, I read a collection of essays by George Orwell. And, although on the surface the two were unrelated, I also watched a documentary about Ram Dass on Netflix. Ram Dass, whose real name was Richard Alpert, was an apostle of LSD in the 1960s, along with Timothy Leary. Later on he became a guru of mindfulness and apparently had a huge following. A stroke left him paralyzed on one side, but also, he explains, even more serene and benevolent than before, even more alert to the splendors of the world. He congratulates himself in a voice as meek as a friar's, as if steeped in ecstasy. So here we have—at least as far as he's concerned—someone who's achieved the state of wonder and serenity that art, according to Glenn Gould, aims to construct. Watching this documentary, I imagined the sarcasm, and even the disgust, that Ram Dass—although probably not Glenn Gould, who was an eccentric and asocial genius—would have inspired in Orwell: this sententious old man, this exemplary representative of the tribe of bearded, vegetarian, sandal-wearing yogis Orwell believed weren't just harmless twits, but malicious idiots to boot. And, looking at these tree-hugging youths in their Peruvian beanies, I also wonder: How is it that the accent of truth, the weight of experience, and even aesthetic enjoyment are so obviously on Orwell's side, and not on that of Ram Dass or any of the self-proclaimed spiritual masters who prattle on about expanding your awareness, the power of the present, and inner peace? Why are these thoughts so lacking in gravitas? Why do they fail the test of beauty so miserably? Why are these books with pink or sky-blue covers, which jump out at you like the incense in New Age bookshops, so ugly, and so stupid?

Taming buffaloes

It's only the second day, but the space allotted to us has become our world, like the monk's quarters, the convict's cell, the buffalo's pen. That's a classic metaphor, the buffalo in its pen. It symbolizes the mind: powerful, capable of great tasks, but also wild, impulsive, perpetually charging off in all directions. It must be tamed. That takes time, patience, skill. We let the buffalo run wild in its pen, then, tirelessly, we bring it back to its post. At the end, the trainer holds the buffalo by its halter and the buffalo obediently follows where he leads. The vritti are stilled, the mind is under control, deliverance is in sight. In Buddhist countries, many popular illustrations represent the stages of this training. They tell us that it's a well-known, well-defined process, and that if we persevere, we'll succeed. They tell us that meditation works. That yoga works. We believe it, otherwise we wouldn't be here.

Screwing in the woods

Busy as we are domesticating the buffaloes in our enclosure, we've all but forgotten that there are other buffaloes nearby, within earshot, in an enclosure just across the way. A parallel, symmetrical space, where everything is identical except that its inhabitants are women. On the other side of the hall, which they access through a door in the far wall, are bungalows and dormitories occupied by women. Sometimes, from a distance, through the trees, on fenced-off paths like our own, we see women passing. In the forum discussions about Vipassana, some see this separation of the sexes as a sign of religious obscurantism, the beginning of coercion and fanaticism. I disagree: it's both wise and realistic. If you want people to look inside themselves for a few days, it's better to spare them the temptation of flirting at the same time. What would become of my already faltering concentration if, instead of the reincarnated Mr. Ribotton, an attractive woman was sitting on the cushion next to me? That said, we're forgetting about gay people. All of a sudden I imagine stolen looks between two big mustached guys, who certainly wouldn't have seen this coming. Direct, wild gay seduction: one after the other, they leave the hall a few minutes apart and meet up in the woods to screw to their hearts' content. When they're done, one offers the other a cigarette and later a shot of the whiskey he keeps in his room: adding transgression to transgression. "I've just about had it up to here with their silence, you?" says the guy with the southern accent. They laugh. Suddenly the simple, raw truth of sex and lust makes a mockery of the spiritualistic pretensions they too took so seriously when they arrived. And they're still laughing later on, now a couple, when they tell their friends the story of how they met at the Vipassana session. Everyone knows it, everyone wants to hear it again and again. It's their showpiece, their grand exploit, their golden legend.

So unexpected, so unthinkable, and for that reason all the more glorious: a far cry from meeting on Mykonos, that's for sure. They laugh. I laugh too, imagining them. But I can't help wondering: Isn't meditation's worldview missing something? Isn't its wisdom a little too wise? Isn't screwing simply *truer*?

The wrong path

Apart from the path to escape the human condition, say Patanjali and Hervé, nothing deserves to be known. For me there are days like today when I think that a thousand other things are more worth knowing. That you learn more about life by going into backrooms and doing politics or mergers and acquisitions than you do sitting on a cushion, telling yourself that by observing your breath you're doing the most crucial thing in the world. And that's just what my concentration tells me when I return to my little cushion. I'm distracted, agitated, I no longer believe in what I'm doing. These doubts make me all the more aggressive, and since there's no one else to be aggressive toward, I'm aggressive toward myself. More than aggressive: hostile. I blame myself for being here, I blame myself for being who I am. My upbeat, subtle little book on yoga strikes me as stupid. Without my having seen it coming, my anger turns to fear. Something is swirling and rising in my mind. Something I have no control over: fear. Unreasoned, unformulated fear. The most specific thing I could say about it would be: I'm afraid I took the wrong path. I feel like I took the wrong path. Only I don't know it yet. I tell myself my life is getting better and better, but it's not true. Things seem to be going well, I believe I'm safe in my enclosure, I think I'm heading toward a state of wonder and serenity, but it's an illusion. The feeling of danger grows. As for the story about the woman and the Gemini statue I hold so dear and believe is so good and even so innocent: danger. The Gemini twins themselves warn: danger of duplicity, danger of division, danger of leading a double life. I feel like I've lost my way, gone astray, taken a wrong turn at a crossroads and ventured into a zone where I don't belong. That's it: I am where I don't belong. Where I shouldn't have gone. To curtail the anxiety that's twisting my guts, I try to focus on my breathing: no use. On my nostrils, the inside of my nostrils, the sensations in my nostrils: Are you kidding me or what?

Tears

At this point something strange happens. A memory emerges. No doubt it took a whole chain of vritti for it to burst like a bubble on the surface of my consciousness, but I didn't see it coming. Suddenly it's here, it hits me like a ton of bricks. I'm in eighth grade, in science class. A boy in the front row stretches out his legs, and the soles of his shoes briefly touch Mr. Ribotton's trousers. Mr. Ribotton feels them, the way amid a pressing crowd Jesus feels that a woman has touched his robe. He looks at the hem of his trousers and his face decomposes. He's filled with a terrible fury. This fury inspires neither fear nor respect, more like pity and embarrassment. In a bitter, whining rage, Mr. Ribotton says he's sick and tired of coming to school just to have someone dirty the trousers he has enough trouble buying because everything costs a fortune and he earns next to nothing, and if the parents of the student who's just dirtied his trousers can afford to have their clothes dry-cleaned every day, good for them, but he can't. His voice shakes as he says this, you'd think he was going to cry, and I'm almost crying too, both because of Mr. Ribotton and because of Maxime Ribotton, who has to sit and watch his father humiliate himself in front of us all, and vent with ghastly indecency his resentment at having been so cheated by life. I look over at him, this fat, sweaty boy whom nobody likes. I expect that after this excruciating ordeal he'll silently leave the school at the end of class and that we'll never see him again. I expect we'll find out that he lay down and hasn't got up, that he's stopped speaking and eating. Some of us will visit him, bring him little gifts in an effort to keep him alive, but it won't work. What Maxime Ribotton is going through is so ghastly that he'll never survive. The whole class will attend his funeral. Following his son's coffin, Mr. Ribotton will wear his best-ironed pair of trousers. His immense grief doesn't stop him from being ridiculous, but we swear never to laugh at him again, to

be kind to him always, to spend our Thursday afternoons
consoling him for his loss. In fact, Maxime Ribotton wasn't
particularly put out by what I considered his father's horrible way of humiliating himself. He shrugged it off after
class with a smirk, saying that his father got angry quickly
but then he calmed down quickly too, so no big deal. But
for me it was a big deal, it's never stopped being a big deal.
And forty-five years on, thinking about Mr. Ribotton's trousers, about the people who can afford to have their clothes
dry-cleaned every day and those, like him, who can't and
hate the world for it, all the misery and sadness of the
world comes crashing down on me. I'm no longer almost
crying: I am crying. Tears stream down my cheeks, tears
that will never cease, tears that will flow as long as human
misery exists. The misery of the victims, the misery of the
humiliated, the misery of the washouts, the misery of the
morons, the misery of the poor little Mr. Ribottons who
make up 99 percent of humanity, but also the misery of
the proud like me who believe they are the remaining
1 percent, the 1 percent who rise and grow with the challenges they face, the 1 percent who believe they're on their
way to a state of wonder and serenity and who are generally in for a fall when they least expect it. The misery of
those who have no idea just how miserable they are, the
misery of the mean. The misery of the executioners, who
are no doubt the most miserable of all and who move me
even more than their victims. The misery deeper yet than
that of the tramp: that of the shaved-head shithead who
sets the tramp on fire. The misery of the murderer, the

misery of the pedophile, the misery of the serial killer, the misery of the guy who struggles against his worst impulses and fails, and who knows from the start that he's going to fail. The misery we've all experienced when, sitting on the crapper in the cold, yellow light of a sleepless night, we think about the noble image we desperately try to convey to others, and the horrible truth of what really dwells within us, in the secrecy of our hearts and our crappers. Fear, shame, and hatred: the grand trinity. That's something we all know, otherwise we wouldn't be human, otherwise we'd be fools. However, for some people it's their whole story, the story of their life, and they try to fill this great white void by lying. They lie for twenty-odd years the way Jean-Claude Romand—whose devastating story I spent seven years writing—did, and then they end up massacring their family, wife, children, parents, and dog, because now that we've come this far into the void, that's all there's left to do. The misery of the little boy in a short story by Dino Buzzati, one of the ones that struck such a chord in me as a teenager, called "Poor Little Boy," about an ungrateful, malicious, sad little boy like Maxime Ribotton. He's in a park with his mother, all the other kids make fun of him, bully him, humiliate him, push him away when he wants to play. At the end a lady says to his mother as she leaves: "Well, goodbye, Mrs. Hitler." I keep crying, I'm nothing but tears on my zafu, and then I hear someone sniffling to my right. As I know, to my right is the reincarnated Mr. Ribotton. It's Mr. Ribotton who's sniffling. But this time it's not his noisy breathing, which I'm more or less used to, it's something else. So I do what's not done: not only do I open my eyes, but I turn slightly to look at him, and although I can only see him in profile I can see that big tears are streaming down Mr. Ribotton's cheeks just like they're streaming down mine, and that Mr. Ribotton, with his wine-toned jacquard sweater and pointed goatee, is weeping, weeping, weeping endlessly like me.

Under the banyan tree

This morning at four thirty, it's a pleasure to settle back in on my zafu. I adjust the cushion, drape myself in the warm, soft, protective blanket. There's still time to move, I can try out different positions before choosing the one I'll hold for the next two hours. Out of the corner of my eye I glimpse my neighbors, who are also getting ready for the session to start. I close my eyes and hear knees cracking, blankets rustling, breaths being snatched, throats being cleared: an orchestra tuning up. I focus on the sounds, isolate them, distinguish between them, my hearing becomes attuned. Finally, the voice emerges from the silence: an ancestral voice, a voice like a centuries-old banyan tree in whose roots a whole village can shelter. You never know how long the invocation will last. It can be five minutes, it can be twenty, it can be followed by instructions or not. It's good to be borne along by this voice that's so deep, that's come so far, that's so free from haste and unrest. Then comes the moment when it stops, and the silence returns. It's funny, now I can sense when it will happen. A few seconds beforehand, I sense that S. N. Goenka will withdraw and leave us alone. He'll be back, don't worry. We're not worried. We're fine.

We're fine

Fortunately, I also know other ways to be fine. Having sex with a woman I love, eye to eye. Swimming in the sea, for a long time. Watching my children—and now my grandson—grow up. Working, when I can. But when it's good, the experience of meditation is an unconditional way to be fine. You're fine because you're here. You're fine because nowhere are you better than you are when you're here. In this body, posted calmly on the border between yourself and the world, between the inside and the outside, and feeling yourself living. Not doing something: simply living. It's nothing extraordinary, quite the opposite: it's the ordinary itself. Life flows inside you like the blood in your veins. Normal, banal—only a little disconnected from the words we use to describe it. When you enter this ordinary state, you say to yourself that it's so simple, so normal, that you should be able to come back to it at any moment. It's always there, you just have to be there too. It's a room inside you, you just have to push open the door to go inside. You

know the way, you have the key, you should be able to come
back whenever you want. Wrong: just because it's inside
you doesn't mean you can go inside. The room is still there,
yes, and there's nothing simpler than entering it. Only: you
can't go in whenever you want to because while it is simple, you are not. It's unchanging, you change. Whenever I
thought I could enter this simple, normal, ordinary state
at will, whenever I thought I'd located and safeguarded
the entrance to the room, I was immediately kicked out.
Another experience of meditation that's as basic as it is
banal: what you want to grab hold of escapes you the very
moment you try. Meaning that this ordinary state, so beneficial, so desirable, is—at least for people like me—of very
short duration. But knowing that it exists, that a practice
that's at first sight outlandish will let you enter it from time
to time—not anytime you want or on command, but quite
often—is invaluable. It changes your life. The voice starts
up again. You get the feeling it's rising from the depths of
yourself, from a cave deep within you, and not from a loud-
speaker. The sutra starts, you don't know how long it will
last but the fact that it's starting means that the session is
almost over. Most of the time this is good news. We can
hardly take it anymore, it hurts everywhere, our only desire
is to uncross our legs, stretch, go for a walk, drink bagged
tea out of a Pyrex glass and eat a prune—which is what
passes for breakfast here. But sometimes, like this morning, we want it to last longer. We want this timeless voice
to never stop rolling its rounded, raspy syllables like peb-
bles in the surf, enemies to all change. We'd like it to last
forever. We're fine.

The great law of alternation

S. N. Goenka warned us: the second day is generally difficult. It's the same when you hike. On the second day you're
stiff, your feet are blistered, your thighs burn as you go
down the steps of the hut, you wonder why you're doing
this, why, when nothing's forcing you to inflict such punish-
ment on yourself. And then the next day off you fly, heartily attacking the slopes that only the day before would have
demolished your legs, you're ready to skip the pause and do
two stages in one. An intensive meditation workshop is like
a hike, which itself is like life: there are stages; landscapes
that change depending on the altitude, sun, and rain; good
days and bad days. Today I feel good on my cushion. Yesterday was horrible. Yesterday I didn't think I'd make it. I
was sure I'd have to call it quits. Yesterday besides worrying, I hated myself, meaning I attached way too much
importance to myself—but this is what I think today. I'm
changeable, we're changeable, the world is changeable. The
only thing that will never change is the fact that everything
changes, all the time. That's what the *I Ching* and all of
Chinese thought say. And not just the Chinese: Plato also
says it in the *Phaedo*, as does the book of Ecclesiastes—"A
time to be born, a time to die, a time to love, a time to
hate . . ."—as well as simple common sense: good weather
follows the rain. Only, the Chinese understood it better
than all the rest. At the heart of their thought is the great
law of alternation, which holds that all of life's phenomena
go by twos and are generated reciprocally: day and night,
storm and calm, empty and full, joy and sadness, opening

and closing, life and death, plus and minus, attack and
parry, war and peace, cold and hot, rest and movement,
breathing in and breathing out, Alex and Alan . . . You can
go on forever like that, and when I get started it's hard to
stop me, as the journalist who came to interview me on
meditation—the one who gave me the idea of writing my
upbeat, subtle little book on yoga—noticed. Seeing that he
was unfamiliar with the notions of yin and yang, I put my
all into explaining to him that that's what the Chinese call
the two forces, poles, or modalities of being without which
there would be no cosmos, no life, nothing at all. Any situation, any state of the world or the mind is a combination
of yin and yang: a changing, transitory combination that's
always evolving toward another combination. A yin force is
destined to become a yang force, and vice versa, like night
becomes day and day becomes night. The day tends toward dusk, the night toward dawn, yin is yang in the making, yang is nascent yin, and we are caught in the current
of this never-ending metamorphosis. It's pointless to resist
it, but it's useful to see it for what it is—and it's sometimes
possible to anticipate it. Knowing that any given moment is
a passage, that a climax announces decline and that a defeat announces victory, can help you live. When life smiles
on you, it's useful to know that it's going to give you a real
thrashing, and when you grope in the darkness, that the
light will return. It makes you cautious and gives you confidence. It helps put your moods in perspective. At least it
should.

Both are true

I say "it should" because in fact if there's one thing I find hard to bear, it's this grand lesson that I endlessly try to hammer home to myself. Not just because I don't know how to put my moods in perspective. It's also because when things are going well, I expect that at one time or another they'll take a turn for the worse—in which I'm right—whereas when things are going badly, I can't believe that at some point they'll take a turn for the better—in which I'm wrong. It's what's called having a gloomy disposition, seeing the glass as half empty rather than as half full. Every negative thought that crosses my mind and fills me with anxiety during a sleepless night when I'm down in the dumps, I think is *truer* than what I think when life seems beautiful, open and auspicious. I'm convinced it's the truth, the bottom line, and that my moments of confidence are illusions. Generally speaking, I think the night is right. "Joy is deeper still than grief can be," Nietzsche tells us. I ask nothing better than to believe it, but at a deeper level, in the depths that make us what we are and over which we have no control, like Van Gogh, I think that "sadness will last forever," and that sadness knows more about life than joy does. Meditation is also here to teach us that both are true, that sadness is as true as joy, joy as true as sadness. In the meantime, today I'm doing just fine.

Up the embankment

Up a little embankment beside the path there's a white plastic garden chair. It took me some time to pluck up the courage to approach it, as if the fact that no one was sitting on it meant that it was forbidden to sit on it at all. Finally, on the midafternoon walk, I went for it. After checking to make sure that no one was coming down the path, I climbed up the small slope, wiped the wet seat with the sleeve of my parka, and when I sat down the legs of the chair sank a good four inches into the mud and dead leaves. Sitting there, I felt that I'd found my place. You could say that on a meditation retreat everyone's place is on their zafu. And if you want to be even cleverer, you could say that everyone's place is *where they are*, no matter where that is. But if you're an old urban hippie like me, you can also say what Don Juan, the shaman who initiated Carlos Castañeda into the mysteries of Yaqui magic, says: everyone has a place on earth that is theirs, a place that is *their place*. Some know theirs and occupy it, others don't: their destinies are not the same. Right then I knew that for the rest of the retreat, that wobbly old plastic chair, stained by humidity, would be mine.

"Words, words, words . . ."

From my embankment you get a view that you'd never suspect from down on the path, over a rain-soaked field on the edge of the woods, over the narrow, oak-lined road that leads to the retreat, and, beyond it, out over the damp gray countryside. It's almost weird getting a glimpse outside the enclosure. Something wriggles under the loose brown earth on the field below: a mole? What else could it be? I don't know how long I sat there on my plastic chair, sunk halfway into the mud, watching the earth wriggling and the mole wriggling beneath it. Maybe five minutes, maybe an hour. In any case I felt good, and I think that those five minutes or that hour watching the earth and the mole wriggling was the first real moment of meditation in the three days that I've been sitting on my zafu and focusing on the inside of my nostrils. Of course as soon as I think that it's over, the merry-go-round starts up once again. Nevertheless, it turns slower. The horses revolve in slow motion, like the rides I took in my childhood where you had to hook metal rings with a stick: I loved that. It's thoughts like these that cross my mind, like birds whizzing through the air. Sweet, peaceful thoughts, thoughts in tune with

the gray, rainy sky. On the one hand I get a certain sense
of satisfaction from them, but at the same time they make
me a little sad, because I realize that something wonderful
will always remain inaccessible to me. A quiet moment like
this, a moment that could be contemplative, a moment I
could just experience, I can never really experience; I can
never live, simply live, because right away I feel the need to
put it into words. I don't have direct access to experience,
I always have to put it into words. I'm not saying that's
bad. It's my reason for being, it's why I'm here, and I'm not
complaining, I'm terrifically lucky to have what's known as
a vocation. But all the same, how good it would be, how
restful it would be, what a huge step forward it would be,
if I could make fewer sentences and see a little more. If I
could see things as they are, instead of pasting this vision
over with the sort of nonstop, subjective, wordy, one-sided,
narrow commentary that we produce all the time without
even being aware of it. This constant inner babbling gets on
my nerves. I don't like it at all. I'd like to think something
other than what I think, because what I think—which I've
catalogued so many times—is vain, repetitive, and pathetically self-centered. I wish I had more worthy thoughts,
thoughts I could be proud of, altruistic thoughts, for example. I'd like to be a good man, a man devoted to his fellow
men, I'd like to be someone people can rely on. Instead I'm
a narcissistic, unstable man, obsessed with being a great
writer. But that's my lot, my baggage, you have to work with
the available material, and it's in this fellow's skin and no
one else's that I have to make the crossing. If only I could
feel more relaxed in his company. If only I could see in

this guy who's so caught up with his own complications the poor little boy that he still is deep down. And if only, instead of dragging him over the coals or erecting statues in his honor, I could console him, cry over him and cry with him, the way I cried with Mr. Ribotton.

William Hurt

Thirty-five years ago, when I was a young journalist, I interviewed the American actor William Hurt. He was at the start of an exceptional career, aided by his physique, his presence, and above all his soft, husky, incredibly captivating voice, and he impressed me no end. Sitting at the bar of a grand Parisian hotel, he wore sandals and Brazilian bracelets, and looked like one of those long-distance travelers you meet in Asia who's always got fascinating stories to tell. He fielded with good grace the inevitable questions about his latest roles and the directors he'd worked with. Nevertheless I felt he'd rather be talking about something else: life, the meaning of existence, the mirage of human identity. I didn't see it at the time, but looking back I think he meditated. He looked like the sort of guy who meditated. I can spot them now, I had the same feeling when I met David Lynch. For a quarter of an hour, William Hurt had been telling me about his efforts to become a better person. Young and dumb as I was, I took on the amused look of someone who's not taken in by virtuous speeches, and asked him why he cared so much about becoming a better person. Then he cut me to the quick. He looked at me, I mean really looked at me, as if for the first time since the start of our meeting, and probably since the start of his interviews that day, someone was asking him a real question. The pupils of his blue eyes widened, he leaned toward me, and he whispered, almost in my ear, "Because it makes you a better actor."

The thief

Years have passed, and today I could say what William Hurt said. What I try to do in life is become a better person—a little less ignorant, a little freer, a little more loving, a little less burdened by my ego, for me that's all the same thing. And I try to become a better person because it'll make me a better writer. What comes first? What's my real goal? On good days, I tell myself that the two are like horses harnessed together—and I remember that that's the original meaning of the word *yoga*: the yoke with which we harness two horses or buffaloes. On less good days, I feel like an impostor. I write to become a better human being, it's true, I write because I love writing, I write because I like to see a job well done, I write because it's my way of knowing reality. I also write to be famous and admired, which is certainly not the best way to become a better person. My work is the cornerstone of my ego. That said, I think there's no reason to dig too deep or ask too many questions about the purity of one's intentions. A story I love says that very well. One day a thief heard about a treasure that some monks were keeping in a hidden room in their monastery. Hoping to get his hands on it, he entered the monastery as a hired hand. For ten years he swept the yard, collected the rubbish, performed the humblest tasks, all the while snooping around, eavesdropping on the monks to try to find out where the treasure could be. After ten years, he'd put so much energy into satisfying his greed that the abbot offered him a position as a novice. He served his novitiate for another ten years, still spying and nosing around, more obsessed with the treasure than ever. Ten more years passed and he was ordained, and he prayed day after day, still hoping to find the treasure and make off with it. In this way he became a great saint, and it's only at the end of his life, on his deathbed, that he understands that the treasure was just that: his life in the monastery, his prayers, his relations with the brothers, and that if he acceded to it, it was because he was a thief. When I criticize myself too much for my foul character, when I complain too much about my self-centeredness, this story is a great comfort to me.

The wolf

Another memory of journalism from around the time when I was attending the Dojo de la Montagne in the early nineties: I'd been commissioned by a magazine to do a story on crossing Canada by train—certainly the least grueling report I've ever written. This sort of transcontinental train is the land equivalent of a cruise ship. It carries neither goods nor real passengers, but almost exclusively elderly, well-off couples celebrating their silver or golden anniversaries. I was the only one traveling alone, no one talked to me, I didn't talk to anyone. The only choices I had to make were between the first and second service in the restaurant car, and whether I'd watch the scenery from the Panorama car or from my spacious, cozy cabin, which—I'm not making this up—even had a bathtub. The hours passed in a cottony torpor. The train's shock absorbers were so smooth that you had to look out the window to see if you were

moving or standing still, and even that wasn't always sufficient because the landscape itself was often so flat and
white that it seemed frozen. I dozed a lot. Sitting on my
zafu—which at that time I took everywhere, although a
folded blanket would have done just as well—I practiced
the small circulation—saving the large circulation for later.
Oh, yes! I did have another decision to make. The crossing
from Montreal to Vancouver takes four days, but you can
get off wherever you like, stay as long as you want, then
take the next train whenever you feel like it. Having no
compelling reason to stop in Saskatoon rather than Winnipeg, to choose where to get off I relied either on the *I Ching*
or on the travel guide's descriptions of what each stop had
to offer. "Here in Canada," the Canadians say, "we might
not have a history but we sure do have geography." Lacking
monuments or remarkable sites, these large prairie towns
all try to appear one way or another in *The Guinness Book
of World Records*. While one boasts the largest swimming
pool in the world, the next has the highest TV tower, and
Winnipeg—again I'm not making this up—prides itself on
having the "windiest street corner in the world." I didn't
have much material for my story, so I went there, and all I
can tell you is that this street corner is windy, sure, but *not
as windy as all that*. After spending an hour there I could
say that with some certainty. However, I did spend two
days at a rather posh winter resort in the Rocky Mountains. As the magazine had an agreement with the hotel
chain, I found myself in a grand hotel that was an exact
replica of the Overlook Hotel in *The Shining*. I was given a
room on the second floor, a few doors down from room 237,

which, as any Kubrick fan will know, is the epicenter of
the horrors that beset Jack Nicholson and his family. My
first impulse, no sooner had I settled in, was to walk down
the hallway fitted with a carpet with distressing brown and
orange patterns—exactly the same as in the film—stand
in front of room 237, and wait for someone to go in or come
out. I stayed there for almost as long as I stayed at the
windiest street corner in the world, but no one went in or
came out, the door remained closed, the horrors remained
unleashed. Whether it was to distract me from room 237
or to curry favor with the magazine that sent me, the hotel
management showered me with bottles of champagne, bas-
kets of fruit, and invitations to the spa. Needless to say, it
was a little disheartening to enjoy all this luxury alone with
my zafu. Rather than a companion, I was offered a ski in-
structor. I ski badly but I had nothing else to do, so I said
fine, why not? Not long afterward, a guy with a silky white
beard knocks on my door, dressed in a red ski suit with
white trim—so pretty much done up as Father Christmas.
On the slopes, he does his best to improve my style, and at
one point, trying to get me to grip the snow with my skis,
he says, "It's too bad you don't do tai chi, because this little
movement—here, see?—is just like a movement in tai chi."
"But I do do tai chi!" I exclaim. Father Christmas's blue
eyes light up, and at the end of the lesson we agree to get
together the next morning to practice down by the lake—
because the hotel is on a lake. So that's where we meet
at dawn, dressed in sweatpants, anoraks, and wool hats,
in front of the rather large frozen lake, encircled by snow-
covered pine trees. A wooden dock juts out over the ice,

and that's where we start practicing the form. It's very cold, the moon is just setting, and the sun is beginning to rise behind the pines in a dazzlingly pure sky. Steam comes from our mouths, snow crystals crunch under our feet. Together with the first birdsong, this is the only sound we hear. Like me, Father Christmas practices the Yang style, we're both in our element, perfectly synchronized—well, quite well synchronized—and then he starts doing cloud hands, the movement with which the small woman in our class fended off her attackers in the metro, except that instead of sweeping the air and bringing his two hands in front of him, he suddenly does something completely unexpected, something I at first think must be a variant I'm unfamiliar with, which consists in pointing his finger in my direction, over my shoulder. When the master points at the moon, a Zen proverb says, the astute disciple looks at the moon, while the less astute disciple looks at the master's finger. I behave like the astute disciple and look at what Father Christmas is pointing at, and what he's pointing at is a wolf. A real wolf, gray and white, very handsome, sitting there quietly on its haunches in the snow, its forelegs stretched out in front of it, between the edge of the frozen lake and the white pines. About twenty yards away, I'd say. I understood what Father Christmas didn't need to say: we should not only be silent, but also continue what we're doing because *it interests the wolf.* So we continue, on our dock, with one movement transforming into another, seamlessly, smoothly, without jerks or needless gestures. It flows. It's fluid. In my entire life I've never done and will no doubt never do the form of tai chi the way we did it that morning: in a peacefully uncoiled thread that tamed the wolf. When I say that in thirty years of meditation, tai chi, yoga, et cetera, I've never had an experience that lifted me off my feet it's not true: I saw the light at the Hotel Cornavin, and I did the form of tai chi with the wolf, two moments of rapture that, each in their own way, were every bit as good as teleportation. I don't know how long this one lasted, or rather yes, I do have an idea because the form served as an hourglass: four, maybe five minutes. At the end of these four or five minutes, the wolf got up and, unhurried, returned to the forest, and was immediately swallowed up by the pines. As for us, we continued until the end.

II

1,825 DAYS

"Serious things have happened in our country"

My memory of that scene is very visual, very precise. Waiting for the next meditation session after the late-afternoon break, I lie on my bed and think about my book. The bit with the wolf will make a good chapter. Maybe even a good ending: open and poetic. Ending a book isn't easy. With what image, what idea of life do we want to leave the reader? What meaning do we want to give to the story we've just told? Despite everything, however, I still fall into extremes: bold or blue, enthusiastic or entropic, open or closed. Either the story ends well or it ends poorly. I want it to end well. May my book end well, may my life end well. I think that's what's going to happen. I believe it. Night has fallen. It's raining. It's raining hard. I haven't turned on the light or pulled down the blind, and I look out the window at what it frames: a rectangle of dripping tar. Suddenly a man with an umbrella blocks my view. He came not from the left, not from the right, not from the bottom. He's there, and he's knocking on the window. In this setting where it's forbidden to speak to a soul, this is an absolute transgression. My serenity instantly collapses. As I get up to open the door I'm already thinking: something terrible has taken place. "What's going on? What's happened?" I ask the man. "You have to come with me," he answers. He's one of the helpers, he doesn't seem used to dealing with this kind of situation. Another pointless exchange follows, me asking what's going on, he telling me I have to come with him, I'll find out. Shoes, parka, I join him outside. He holds his umbrella over me as we walk toward the central building. My thoughts are spinning, I wonder who's died. I wonder whose death would devastate me the most. I remember the phone call I got from Catherine, my uncle Nicolas's wife, to tell me that their son François had just committed suicide, and, as she said these words, how Nicolas, who was standing next to her, howled with grief. In a few moments I'll be the one howling. In a few moments my life will be turned upside down, and not at all as I imagined in my absurd dream of wonder and serenity. We go around the building to a side door, where the helper folds his umbrella and shakes it carefully several times before leading me down a dark hallway into a small room cluttered with chests and old furniture, the kind of room where farmers store their personal items once they've turned their farmhouse into a lodge or bed-and-breakfast. We're behind the scenes, where the masks fall. No more Noble Silence, no more playacting, no more fun. Standing in front of the window in sweatpants and a fleece jacket is the tall, thin guy with the protruding Adam's apple whom I've never seen do anything but sit cross-legged on the platform, draped in a blue blanket, watching silently over our meditation. The jerk could have come to my room to say what he's got to say instead of sending this catatonic gonad, I think to myself. I ask what's going on, what happened. "Don't worry," he told me, "it's no one in your family, no one very close to you. But you should know that in the past few days serious things have happened in our country."

A drive through the night

In the end it was the taxi driver who set me straight. The thin guy at the retreat had been vague, evasive, less to spare my feelings, I think, than because he neither knew nor cared much about what had happened. He'd written down the two things he had to tell me on a piece of paper: *Charlie Hebdo*—as if he needed the reminder so as not to forget the magazine's name—and, a little further down: Bernard . . . Maris . . . He had trouble reading his own handwriting, and the name was no doubt unfamiliar to him. I have to be honest, and I'm sure I'll be understood: I felt huge relief to learn that it was Bernard who'd died in a terrorist attack and not someone closer, not one of my children. While his superior returned—I assume—to his cushion, the helper checked the time of the last train to Paris and called a taxi to take me to Migennes. The drive lasted three quarters of an hour and took place entirely in the dark. The villages were unlit, the road was unlit, and not a single car passed us going the other way. Having made the trip in the opposite direction, I knew that we were crossing forests and passing ponds, but you couldn't see a thing. Everything was engulfed in darkness, as if the power in the entire region had been cut by a disaster and we risked being attacked by zombie farmers at any moment. I sat in the front next to the driver. He was a stocky guy around my age with a mustache and a friendly face, who didn't stop talking the whole way and from whom I learned, for starters, of the deaths of the cartoonists Cabu and Wolinski. Cabu and Wolinski! Cabu and Wolinski, who'd been part of my adolescence, when Emmanuel Guilhen and I read *Charlie Hebdo*. Cabu and Wolinski, of whom I'd since lost sight, as I'd lost sight of all my teenage friends, as I'd lost sight of Emmanuel Guilhen. And I don't know what astonished me the most: to learn that Cabu and Wolinski had been murdered by Islamist terrorists, or to discover that they were both a good eighty years old. Another thing that was perhaps not astonishing but that surprised me all the same was the familiarity with which this taxi driver from the Morvan region talked not only about Cabu and Wolinski, but also about the other murdered cartoonists, although I was learning only now both of their existence and of their death. Four days earlier he'd had no idea who they were, or what *Charlie Hebdo* was for that matter. But now it was as if, retroactively, he'd been reading the magazine all his life. As if retroactively since his youth, he'd gone each week to buy it at the kiosk in the Migennes station, where they put it aside for him. And he knew who Bernard Maris was as well. I wanted to ask how he knew so much for someone who didn't listen to the radio. But even as I formed the question in my mind, he politely suggested that we turn it on. Then when he pushed the button it was as if the whole event redoubled in enormity. Demonstrations were bringing together millions of people across France, forty-four foreign heads of state had come to take part in a huge unity march . . . Everyone, absolutely everyone in France knew what had happened, with the exception of the hundred or so people I'd been one of not an hour earlier. The driver wasn't particularly surprised by my ignorance. He drove people to and from the Vipassana center from time to time, and their bizarre practices inspired in him neither suspicion nor mockery, as I would have expected. He knew more or less what meditation was—in any case more than the journalist who'd interviewed me on the subject and given me the idea of writing this book—and I could well imagine him talking about Patanjali with as much fervor as when he talked about Charb or Tignous, cartoonists who were also killed in the attack. When I remarked that I found it strange, all the same, to have spent the past few days glued to a little cushion without knowing that something like the French 9/11 had taken place, he thought for a moment and then gave me a no-nonsense answer for which I'm still grateful: "If you'd known, what would it have changed?"

Hélène and Bernard

A little while ago I mentioned my friend Hélène F., who starts most of her sentences with "You" rather than "I." She works for a magazine dedicated to wellness, personal development, and disseminating a positive vision of life according to which, in a nutshell, the worst thing that can happen to you is actually a boon: a chance to develop and become better. In it there's a lot of talk of yoga, meditation, and mindfulness. I like Hélène's take on her work and the things it deals with: she jokes about them while taking them seriously at the same time. Although she's aware of how caricatural this doctrine can seem, she fully subscribes to the worldview that underlies it, and I quite agree with her. This openness also makes her a precious friend when times are tough: she listens, and always finds something fitting to say. Two years earlier, she was the one who'd needed help when she went through a harrowing divorce. The whole time she maintained a sense of integrity, practicality, and good cheer, but although she didn't go as far as thinking that at forty her love life was over and done with—such melodrama isn't her style—she did think it would be a long time before she regained the desire and strength to love. It was then, when she believed that love was out of the question, that she fell in love. Head over heels, she said. She talked a lot about the man she'd fallen head over heels in love with, in fact she no longer talked about anything else. However, she didn't tell us either his name or his profession or to which world he belonged, because although he wasn't married he'd been widowed very recently, he was quite well known, and for the moment their affair was a secret. This constraint didn't bother Hélène, who on principle never asks people *what they do*, because she finds out soon enough and because it's above all *who they are* that interests her. Her lover's social persona thus under wraps, all she told us about was the enchanted tête-à-tête their lives had become since the day they met, peppering her account with the banal phrases that are, I believe, the sign of true love: "It's as if we were made for each other . . . I think of him all the time, I know he thinks of me all the time . . . We get along so well . . . You know, it's as if I were in love for the first time . . ." Such an encounter is the best thing that can happen to someone. Many people have to go through life without experiencing anything like it, and those who do experience it—I don't know the percentage, but let's say it's around 20 percent of the population, which is no more or less arbitrary than saying that the brain is focused on the present 20 percent of the time—are the only truly happy people in the world. When life gives you such a blessing you have to seize it and hold it tight, because there's nothing more precious, and few things can measure up to it. And if you're unfortunate or stupid enough to miss out on it, life after such an error is bound to be bitter and unpleasant—a subject I could go on about for some time. One evening, Hélène brought Bernard over to our place for dinner. It was the first time they'd gone out together—I mean the first time they'd shown themselves to the world, if you can call our home the world. For the first time they were escaping their enchanted tête-à-tête to have dinner with other people, and that night it felt good to be the "other people." It was good to witness the continuous sense of wonder they felt, to see them looking at each other, listening to each other, and it was also good to be in the same room as Bernard. You didn't have to be in love with him to find him immediately—and remarkably—lovable. He had the handsome face of an American actor, a big, toothy smile and a slight Toulousian drawl, he was a good talker but he also knew how to be silent, and his silences had a way of putting you at ease. A professor of economics, he was well known for his weekly radio program and his regular appearances on TV. I almost always agreed with him when he talked about economics—which I don't understand at all—because he said I was right not to understand and that that was precisely the point: we're not supposed to understand it because it's nothing but obfuscation in the service of the rich. Every Friday morning he had a ritualized radio spat with a neoliberal journalist across from whom he played the role of the Red. Only he

was a funny kind of Red, because while he was a key figure in the alter-globalist movement ATTAC, he was also
a member of the General Council of the Bank of France.
It's a trait that I got to know and like about him: his way
of having a foot in every camp, in every caste, moving
among as many different milieus as possible. The offspring
of Toulousian anarchists, he'd married the daughter of a
member of the ultra-elite Académie Française and lived in
a luxurious apartment in Paris's Sixteenth Arrondissement
that had belonged to her, while at the same time hanging
out with the iconoclastic, foul-mouthed gang of journalists
and cartoonists at *Charlie Hebdo*. There he wrote about
economics, but also more and more about literature. In fact
he loved literature above all else, and that's basically all
we talked about during the—what?—five or six times we
had dinner together. We were in no hurry, we were slowly
becoming friends, we had time.

Force majeure

The rule at the Vipassana retreat is that your loved ones
may contact you only in a case of force majeure. The attack
was a terrible thing, Bernard's death was a terrible thing,
nevertheless the fact was that he wasn't a close friend and,
as the taxi driver said, it didn't change anything, whether
I knew or not, whether I was in Paris or not, and so it was
not a case of force majeure. Things changed on January 11,
2015, when, while four million French people took to the
streets to mourn the staff of a small satirical magazine

that most of them, like the taxi driver, hadn't even known existed until a couple of days before, Bernard's relatives began organizing his funeral. It was fixed for the fifteenth, in his native village near Toulouse. Hélène and he had been together for just over two years, she was aware that she'd play only a small role at the ceremony vis-à-vis Bernard's official family, but she wanted something else. She wanted someone to talk about Bernard's love of literature—that is, concretely, she wanted a writer whom Bernard liked, and who liked Bernard, to say a few words. Ideally it should have been Michel Houellebecq, about whom Bernard had written a book and with whom he was friends. But once again, Houellebecq was at the heart of the turmoil. His new book, *Submission*, described a France that had converted to Islam en masse. Hélène, Bernard, and I had read it before it appeared, each had reviewed or had to review it, she for *Psychologies* magazine, Bernard for *Charlie*, me for *Le Monde*, and at our last dinner together, ten days before the attack, that was pretty much all we talked about. My article was enthusiastic, but as Hélène mischievously pointed out, even if I weren't all that enthusiastic about it I'd never criticize Houellebecq for fear of appearing jealous—which to be honest, I am. And that's one of the benefits of meditation, we concluded: that you can admit to such a disreputable trait without making a big thing of it. *Submission* appeared on January 7. That is, on the morning of January 7 there were practically no other books in the French bookshops, and practically no other subjects were discussed in the French media. And it was also on January 7, at 11:20 a.m., that two hooded men armed with

Kalashnikovs burst into the newsroom at *Charlie Hebdo* on the second floor of a modern, dreary little building on Rue Nicolas Appert near Place de la République, killed twelve people, and seriously injured five more. Needless to say, some have seen *Submission* as a provocation to which the shooting was a response. Houellebecq was once again put under police protection, his publisher announced that he wouldn't be promoting his book and that he'd be lying low for a time. I came second on the list of Bernard's writer friends. The situation was clear now, a case of force majeure had been established. I could make myself useful, so it was decided that I'd be exfiltrated. That was no small feat. With exasperating calm, the man with the protruding Adam's apple repeated what we'd been told the first day, that Vipassana is like an operation on the depths of the mind, and that it's very dangerous to interrupt it. Besides, he went on, was an interruption really justified? Was it really that serious? Was the murdered friend as close as all that? Couldn't someone else speak at his funeral? The way he asked these questions it wasn't quite as if he'd never heard of the *Charlie Hebdo* attack, but rather as if it had taken place in Syria or the Gaza Strip: fifty people including children killed by rocket fire is terrible, but hey, life can't stop as a result or it'd stop all the time. It's the plain truth: life in general and meditation sessions in particular can't stop every time a catastrophe takes place in the world, otherwise they'd stop all the time. Fine, it's the plain truth, it's common sense, nonetheless it reminded me of the Ayurvedics.

The Ayurvedics

Exactly ten years and seven days earlier, I was spending the Christmas holidays with my family in a coastal village in Sri Lanka that was devastated by the tsunami. I've told all that in another book, here I'd just like to evoke one almost comical detail that took place at the same time as the disaster. One wing of the hotel where we were staying was occupied by a group of Swiss Germans who'd come on a retreat to practice yoga and Ayurvedic healing. The room where they did their exercises was in a separate annex, they ate their meals apart from everyone else, we hardly saw them at all. They were like peripheral silhouettes, wearing white bathrobes, and—don't ask me why—some sort of plastic hygienic caps on their heads. We could hear them from a distance, chanting their mantras. When the wave hit, sweeping away everything in its path, and thousands of people died or went missing, our hotel, protected by its location on the top of a hill, became a disaster refuge, an emergency facility, a psychological support center, a raft of the *Medusa*. Anyone with nowhere to go ended up there. We became particularly attached to a young French couple. They'd lost their four-year-old daughter and were searching for her body in all the morgues along the coast, where the corpses that no one knew what to do with were piling up. We helped them as best we could, and God knows, we weren't the only ones. All those who like us had been spared did their best to care for those who hadn't been so lucky. Everyone was helping, everyone gave what they could, everyone did what they could, it was even uplifting to behold—and reassuring about human nature. Everyone, that is, except the Ayurvedics, who continued to care for their bodies and souls as if nothing had happened, as if nothing was going on around them. We continued to see them on the far side of the terrain, in their bathrobes and swimming caps, walking slowly and, I suppose, mindfully. We continued to hear their mantras, carried by the warm, tropical breeze, extolling the power of the present and the grace of compassion.

The Russian pimp coat

Hélène, whom I went to visit the following morning, was calm and focused—later she told me that I was calm and focused too. I gave her a hug, and then we sat down to talk. It wasn't just a conversation between friends but a business discussion as well, which made things easier for both of us. She had to help me write the best speech I could for Bernard's funeral. I took notes, in a handsome black Moleskine-style notebook I'd been given at one book fair or another. Without my even having to ask, Hélène began to navigate between memories of her two years together with Bernard and memories of the five days since his death— these two segments of time colliding in sometimes bizarre ways. The first thing she told me—or at least, the first thing I jotted down—was that they didn't spend their last night together. Bernard still lived on Rue de l'Assomption, in the large, upscale apartment where he'd lived with his wife, Sylvie, and where Hélène obviously hated going. He, on

the other hand, liked being at her place on Rue de Belle-
fond in the more modest Ninth Arrondissement, not far
from ours. He would gladly have moved in with her—at
least that's what he said—but she didn't see how she could
fit him into the two-bedroom apartment she'd rented for
herself and her children after separating from their father.
It just wasn't meant for a man, especially a man like Bernard, whose possessions didn't exactly fit into a suitcase.
Red as he was, he owned a lot of things: a lot of books,
a lot of clothes, for example his costly, fur-trimmed Mac
Douglas coat, which he wore the first night he came over
to our place for dinner, and which she gently made fun of,
saying it made him look like a Russian pimp. He also wore
it on the day of the attack, although he no longer had it at
the mortuary where his body was transported a few hours
later. Hélène wondered what had become of it, she would
have preferred him still to be wearing it so it could keep
him warm. It must have been left on a coatrack at *Charlie
Hebdo*'s offices, where it probably remained for some time
after the premises were sealed. Bernard liked nice clothes,
he liked good food and tables with many guests. He liked
to talk rubbish, and he liked it when other people talked
rubbish too. He liked contradictions, and he held to his
own. He loved the moment when, widowed, weakened
by cancer, and not expecting much from life, he met this
pretty, clever blonde who was a good twenty years younger
than him, and who fell in love with him as much as he'd
fallen in love with her. He loved to wake up in the morning with the thought that they were in love, and to turn to
her in bed to tell her just that. He loved the fact that they

never tired of telling and retelling the story of how they met, their story, this love that, from one day to the next, had made their lives so alive. Generally speaking, Hélène said, Bernard loved life, and life repaid him in full. But he was also terribly worried and obsessive. He kept his cards close to his chest, people didn't catch on, but Hélène did. Hélène felt like she knew everything about him, as if now that he was dead, all that he was, all that he had been, existed only in her heart. Who but she, for example, knew about the notebook in which he wrote down his dreams and put a mysterious, incomprehensible number after each date? Only she, Hélène, knew that it was the number of days he had left to live. He'd allotted himself 1,825 as of April 1, 2014. Why 1,825? Hélène didn't know. Curiously, she'd never done the calculation I did for her that morning: 1,825 days is five years on the button, so he'd been planning to die on April 1, 2019. Too optimistic, since he died on January 7, 2015, 1,543 days ahead of schedule. On that day, then, Hélène and he spoke for the last time. They spoke on the phone, since they hadn't spent the night together, then they left, each to their respective magazine. They were to meet up again that evening, and this time he was to stay the night. He said to her, "See you this evening, my love." An hour and a half later she was reduced body and soul to the haunting question "Is he dead?" and three hours after that to the equally haunting question "Did he suffer?" The answer: no. When you get a bullet in the head at close range, you don't suffer. At the mortuary, she didn't understand why they'd put a white cloth over his forehead. She was told: it was a dressing to hide the bullet holes in his temples. She went to see him three times. With each visit she had the impression that he'd shrunk, that he was frailer and grayer on the mortuary table, that he looked less and less like himself. On January 10, an Arab family—women and children mostly—mourned loudly in a neighboring room at the morgue. It was the Kouachi family, someone said to her in a hushed voice. The day before, counterterrorist police had shot dead the brothers Chérif and Saïd Kouachi—who had murdered Bernard and the eleven others at *Charlie Hebdo* three days earlier—in a printing works in the Paris suburbs where they'd taken refuge. Hélène isn't the sort of person who thinks that criminals don't deserve to be mourned by their families, or that executioners and victims belong to two separate humanities. Still, it was bizarre to think that the bodies of the Kouachi brothers lay just a few yards from Bernard's. I thought that, even though I could see myself doing it, it wouldn't go down particularly well for me to show sympathy for the Kouachi brothers' families at Bernard's funeral. I had the information I needed for my speech, so I got up and put on my coat. And it was only when I was leaving that both Hélène and I remembered at the same moment a little scene that had taken place on the doorstep after our last dinner together, ten days before the tragedy. We'd drunk quite a bit. As we were leaving, standing right where we were now in the little entranceway beside the coat stand, where in particular the famous Russian pimp coat that Hélène never missed an opportunity to make fun of was hanging, Bernard and I started joking about whether we should shake hands as we'd done up to then, or kiss each other on the cheek. We wondered when and how exactly the habit of men kissing each other on the cheek—which would have seemed completely ridiculous to us in our distant youths—had spread. Then, finally, we kissed each other on the cheek.

I'm downbeat

My words at Bernard's funeral ended with that kiss on the cheek. I'd put a lot of thought into my speech, I think it was good. In any case it made Hélène happy, that was the main thing. Over the next few weeks I saw her quite often, and I was struck by her calm. Her face was smooth, rested, she seemed weightless. She spoke to Bernard all the time, in a low voice, and Bernard spoke to her all the time. He said to her: "Things will be fine, my love, don't worry, my love, things will be fine," and she said to me in a soft voice with an angelic smile: "I'm a little shaky at the moment, you know." Hélène is a remarkably sane woman, you have to be to know in such circumstances that you're a little shaky, and no doubt you have to come to terms with the fact that you're a little shaky to be able to find your bearings when the time comes. She found her bearings, then she met a man, François, who happens to be one of my oldest friends, and she's doing well. On the face of it, there's no reason for her to reappear in this story. I say that, but so many things I hadn't foreseen—let alone wanted—have appeared and reappeared in this story . . . I then plunged back into my yoga book project, meaning that I wrote down my memories of the Vipassana session while they were still fresh, in as much detail as possible. What you've been reading is a fleshed-out version of this text, which subsequently went through quite a few twists and turns—as you'll see if you keep reading. I felt uncomfortable writing it. I didn't know what to think, I didn't know what I was saying, or rather: I didn't know what *it* was saying. When I was there, I knew that I was going to write everything down as soon as I got out. Consequently, despite all my attempts not to, I spent much of my time on the zafu putting together sentences that relate this experience. However, when you put together sentences that relate an experience, it's difficult not to pass judgment. Perhaps if you're a poet you can: you use words in a different way, you bypass the meaning, poetry is the language that's least incompatible with the nonverbal experience of meditation. The poet and writer Henri Michaux spoke this language fluently. Unfortunately for me, I'm not a poet. My craft, my talent, is narration, and in all circumstances what I want to know is: What's the story? It's the exact opposite of meditation, which—twelfth definition—aims to help you stop telling stories. To dissolve the thick layer of narration, of judgment, of commentary with which people so diligently cover up things as they are. I spent the whole Vipassana session not only putting together sentences, but also asking myself what I thought

of the session: More good than bad? More bad than good?
More like more good than bad. But beyond the merits of
the Vipassana school, what I plan to say—the idea that is
to underpin my story, what readers should take away from
it—is simply that meditation is *good*. That yoga is *good*. I'm
not the first to say it, okay. I simply plan to say it from another starting point, let's say from another part of the book-
shop than the personal development section. I plan to say
not only that yoga and meditation make you feel good, but
that, much more than a hobby or a health practice, they're
a way of being in the world, a way of knowing, a way of
accessing reality worthy of occupying a central place in our
lives. That's what I plan to say, on the basis of my admit-
tedly less than rock-solid experience. Only I find it hard
to say it once I get back from my Vipassana retreat. I no
longer know how to say it. I'm no longer as convinced as
I was. I can't help thinking about the Ayurvedics in their
bathrobes and swimming caps in Sri Lanka, and the terrible sarcasm their indifference and stupidity inspired in
Jérôme, the father of the drowned little girl: "You guys all
right? Found your inner peace? Good for you!" It would
be unfair to level the same criticism at the followers and
organizers of Vipassana. It wouldn't have changed anything
or helped anyone to interrupt the retreat or even to make
an announcement—otherwise, it's true, there'd be no end
to such interruptions. Still: even if I don't blame them, I
have the impression that in a toss-up between the blood
and tears shed in Paris in those days, Bernard's brains on
the linoleum floors of *Charlie Hebdo*'s dingy newsroom, and
Hélène's shattered life—to speak here only of the people

I know—and our conclave of meditators busy focusing on their nostrils and silently chewing their bulgur and gomashio, one experience is simply *truer* than the other. Everything that is real is true, by definition, nevertheless some perceptions of the real have a greater truth content than others, and they're not necessarily the most optimistic. I think, for example, that Dostoyevsky's truth content is greater than that of the Dalai Lama. In short, when it came to my upbeat, subtle little book on yoga, I found myself feeling a little downbeat.

The not particularly nice story about the ascetic Sangamaji

When I spoke to Hervé about these doubts, he told me the story of the ascetic Sangamaji. It appears in an important piece of ancient Buddhist scripture, the *Udana*, but there are no references to it in any recent introductions to Buddhism, which is understandable because it's not particularly nice. The ascetic Sangamaji sits meditating under a tree. Before retiring from the world, he lived with a woman with whom he'd had a child. He abandoned them both for higher achievements, or at least for what he considers to be such. Now living in misery, the woman comes to ask him for help. She shows him their skinny, hungry little boy, and pleads with him. He doesn't answer, doesn't blink, and keeps sitting there cross-legged. She insists. He doesn't come out of his meditation. Finally she sets the child down on the ground, saying, "He's your son, monk. You take care of him," and pretends to leave. Hidden behind a tree, she observes the ascetic and the child. The child cries and cries, it's heartbreaking. The ascetic doesn't look at him, doesn't even budge. He continues to meditate. Disgusted, the woman takes back the child and leaves without a word. What's most disturbing about this story is that it's not presented as an example of the sort of awful callousness and perverted devotion practiced by the Ayurvedics in Sri Lanka. Instead of condemning this ascetic who showed as much sympathy as a frozen potato, as Hervé put it, the Buddha congratulates him: "Sangamaji neither rejoices at her arrival, nor grieves at her departure. This Sangamaji, freed from attachment, him I call a Brahmana." The Buddha isn't speaking lightly: compassion is the vibrant heart of Buddhism. "Should we think, then," concludes Hervé, "that Sangamaji's compassion takes place in grander, brighter spheres, in a secret but supremely effective way that escapes us but which the Buddha perceives?"

"Boobs! Boobs!"

Frustrated that I'd completed only half of the Vipassana retreat, a few months later I decided to do another one, and this time I stayed until the end. It was interesting, but the sense of surprise and mystery that enshrouded the first had dissipated. I'd seen the show, I knew what went on backstage, I was a little bored. I cheated a bit, too, and took notes. From this second session one sentence in particular stays with me, which at least partially answers my big question: What's going on in everyone's mind? I tell it with all the more pleasure as it'll be the last funny thing in this story for some time. On the tenth and last day of the session, the Noble Silence is lifted. The women and men mingle again. We talk, we laugh, we smoke cigarettes. We get to know one another. The silence-induced solemnity dissipates. The speechless, hooded zombies who didn't so much as glance at you become people with jobs, homes, political opinions, coarse or strident laughter. It's a touching moment. We compare experiences. When was it the hardest, when did we almost freak out, when were we on the verge of throwing in the towel? I mixed with a small group of guys in their twenties and thirties. One was in sales, another was a fair-trade winegrower, a third was in catering; you meet all kinds in meditation groups. The young guy who worked in catering, dressed in a green-and-mauve fleece jacket with an earring and a strong southwestern accent, said that at one point for him it had been really tough because no matter how much he tried to focus on his breathing, he always thought about the same damn thing. Ten days nonstop, without any distractions, he'd been stuck there thinking the whole time, absolutely the whole time, about the same thing. And what was that?

"Boobs! Boobs!"

That guy was great.

III

THE STORY OF MY MADNESS

The secret room

What happened at the Hotel Cornavin after the yoga retreat in Morges was too overwhelming not to have a future, as would no doubt have been reasonable. Before we separated, the woman who would later give me the Gemini statue and I agreed on a protocol. Apart from the fact that we both practiced yoga, we knew nothing about each other, and we wouldn't try to find out more. We wouldn't tell each other about our lives. We would only meet, at regular intervals, in a hotel in a provincial town—which was not, I think, the town where she lived. I knew nothing about her husband or partner, about her children if she had any, or about her job. Of course you only need to listen to someone for two minutes to get a fairly precise idea of their level of culture and place in society, and I imagined her more readily, let's say, practicing law than selling fruit and vegetables—my loves, I regret to say, have never led me very far from my own social class. And I was never tempted, for example, to open the Moleskine-style notebook I'd seen in her bag while she was taking a shower. The mystery surrounding our vow of mutual ignorance was much stronger than the associated curiosity. She, too, never said a word that suggested she knew I was a writer, and I believe it's entirely possible that even today, wherever she is, she is unaware of the existence of this book. I don't have an address to send it to, not even a last name. There are no witnesses to our story other than the receptionist at a midrange hotel located on a quiet street in a midsize town. It would never have occurred to us to, say, go to an exhibition or take a walk around the town. We'd go into the room, close the door behind us, and make love. And as we made love we'd go higher and higher, to the point that it frightened us sometimes. We were afraid it would stop, and we were afraid it would continue. We also talked a lot. What can you talk about when you know nothing about the other person? All normal, social topics being set aside, there was nothing else in the room, on the bed, but our bodies and, excuse my language, our souls. I've never known anyone as intimately as I knew this stranger. The Gemini woman loved life, and when I say she loved life I don't just mean what that means for most of us: that she loved *her* life, and loved filling it with beautiful, pleasant things. No, it's *life* she loved, all of life, the life of passersby on the street, the life of ants, she truly loved to see the grass grow. I'll never know what it's like to live like that. For me—who despite every effort to reach a state of wonder and serenity has seen more than my fair share of that dreadful abyss known as depression, or madness—it's already a blessing to have been so close to someone with such a natural gift. Fully absorbed in this passion, I didn't want to see that depression and madness were already there, lying in ambush. I closed my ears to the proverb that's as cruel as it is true: "He who has two women loses his soul. He who has two houses loses his mind." I believed my mind was solid, firmly anchored to my body by love, work, and meditation. I told myself that in having such a well-contained affair, not only did I not run the risk of losing my soul, but I was leading my life wisely: I was wisely forgoing some pleasures in exchange for others. "Wisely? Aren't you exaggerating a bit? Aren't you framing things to suit yourself?" said Hervé when I told him—and only him—about this affair. Okay, maybe not "wisely": already it would be good if it remained secret and didn't do any harm. One night we were hungry, and the receptionist told us about the only place still open in the neighborhood. It belonged to the Entrecôte group of restaurants, which have the merit of closing very late and at which they only serve steaks with fries and a sauce that's the house's well-kept secret. It was there that she told me she'd soon be moving very far away, with her family. It was the first time she'd mentioned her family, and she did it in a deliberately vague way, without telling me, for example, how many children she had or how old they were, and when I asked what she meant by "very far away," she replied just as vaguely: "to the Southern Hemisphere." It was in this restaurant, too, after her announcement, that I expressed the seemingly unrealistic wish that our story would last forever—that is, until one of

us died. As long as it remained secret and never came to
light, nothing stopped it from going on like this for years,
decades even, I said. What did it matter if the Gemini
woman moved to the Southern Hemisphere, as she said:
our secret room would continue to exist. No longer in this
hotel in the French provinces, but in a motel in New Zealand, South Africa, or Tasmania. We wouldn't be able to
meet every two weeks, but I could find a way to come every
six months, once a year at the longest, and so basically
nothing would change. This yearly meeting in a motel in
the Southern Hemisphere—known only to us, belonging
only to us—would remain the most precious thing in our
lives. And from the moment this wish was spoken, at the
Entrecôte restaurant where we were now the last customers, it was immediately clear to both of us that it was not,
as reason told us, a pleasant and inconsequential reverie,
but something possible, absolutely possible. And not just
something absolutely possible: something that would happen. That would really happen, that would happen without
a doubt, that was bound to happen: it was no longer a wish,
it was a certainty. We looked at each other, over our steaks
and red wine, and I told her that one day, in ten years, in
twenty years, we'd remember this evening and say, "You
see? It's happened, and it's going to continue, and it won't
end until one of us dies." She smiled when I said that, and,
watching her smile as the waiters turned the chairs over on
the tables to make it increasingly obvious that they were
just waiting for us to clear out, I started to cry, without
seeing it coming. And a little later, back in our room, I
said to her: "Do you know why I started to cry earlier? Not

because you're going to leave—we'll figure that out—but because I thought that you were going to die. Not in an accident or anything, I mean. Just the self-evident truth that one day, like everyone else, you'll die. I hope it'll be a long time from now, I hope you'll be old, I hope it'll be after me, but no matter when it happens, the world will exist without you. And that's why I cried, because I don't know anyone as alive as you, because to me you're the face of life."

The place where you don't lie

It's probably magical thinking, but I date the start of my meltdown to that night. In assuring the Gemini woman that we *too* would always love each other, that on some distant day in the future we'd look back on our lives and remember this wish that had come true against all odds, I let myself be carried away by sincere enthusiasm, but I also challenged the gods: hubris. In aspiring for unity, I made a pact with division. How much can I tell about this meltdown? How much should I keep to myself? Regarding literature, or at least the sort of literature I practice, I have one conviction: it is *the place where you don't lie*. This is the absolute imperative, everything else is incidental, and I think I've always held to it. What I write may be narcissistic and vain, but I'm not lying. I can quietly affirm, and will be able to quietly affirm on Judgment Day, that I write what crosses my mind, what I think, what I am—all of which is certainly nothing to gloat about—"without hypocrisy," as Ludwig Börne demands. However, Ludwig Börne also

demands that it be written "without fabrication." And although I'm usually ready to go along with that, too, here it's
different. Each book imposes its own rules, rules we don't
set in advance, but rather discover with use. I can't say of
this book what I've proudly said of several others: "It's all
true." While writing it, I have to distort a little, transpose
a little, erase a little. Especially erase, because while I can
say whatever I want about myself, including less flattering
truths, I can't do the same with others. I do not give myself the right, nor do I feel the urge, to give the details of
a crisis that is not the subject of this story. And so I shall
lie by omission, and pass directly to the psychological—
and even psychiatric—consequences that this crisis had
on me, and on me alone. Because precisely that thing
happened that, with age, I was sure would never happen
again. My life, which I believed to be so harmonious, so
well fortified, so conducive to writing an upbeat, subtle little book on yoga, was in fact heading for disaster. And this
disaster did not come from external circumstances, cancer,
a tsunami, or the Kouachi brothers kicking open the door
without warning and massacring everyone with Kalashnikovs. No: it came from me. It came from that powerful,
self-destructive streak I had presumptuously believed I was
cured of, and that raged like never before, driving me forever from my enclosure.

Tachypsychia

It's a word I didn't know: *tachypsychia*. The first time I heard it was also the first time I saw a psychiatrist—a gentle, humane man whom I think of with gratitude. Tachypsychia is like tachycardia, only for mental activity. Your thoughts are erratic, disconnected, unrelenting. They're all over the place. They swirl and scathe. They're vritti, but vritti on overdrive, a vritti storm, vritti on cocaine. That's a good description of my state. Rather than being, as I'd thought, well on my way to taming them and reaching a state of wonder and serenity, I've fallen prey to vritti on the rampage. I'm their captive, bound hand and foot. They drive me mad. And I don't use that word lightly: the purpose of the following pages is to examine it. Ever since I came of age I've thought I was a bit more neurotic than average, which has made my life a bit unhappier than average. But it hasn't prevented me from having periods of remission, the longest of which, almost ten years, is the one whose end I'm recounting here. They say it's only when you're no longer happy that you realize you once were. For me that's not true: for ten whole years I knew I was happy. It did my heart good, I thanked the gods, I thanked love, I thanked my own wisdom, and I wanted to protect that happiness to the extent that I could. And throughout this crisis I continued to want that, only I wanted the opposite as well. I wanted disaster as much as I wanted relief, and I oscillated endlessly, unbearably, from one to the other. It's for that reason that I'm no longer in the office of a psycho-analyst, as has happened to me so often in life, but for the first time in that of a psychiatrist, this gentle, humane man who prescribed high doses of an antipsychotic—although, he assures me, I'm not a psychotic—as well as a thymo-regulator, or mood stabilizer, given to people with bipolar disorder.

Type 2

It's disturbing, at almost sixty years of age, to be diagnosed with an illness that you've suffered from your whole life without it ever being named. Your first reaction is to protest. I protested, insisting that bipolar disorder is one of those notions that are all of a sudden in vogue and get pinned on anything and everything—much like gluten intolerance, which so many people discovered they suffered from as soon as people started talking about it. Then you read what you can on the subject, you reexamine your whole life from that angle, and you realize that the shoe fits. Perfectly, even. That all your life you've been subject to this alternation of excitement and depression that is of course the lot of us all—because all our moods change, we all have highs and lows, clear skies and dark clouds—only that there's a group of people to which you belong, along with, it seems, 2 percent of the population, for whom the highs are higher and the lows lower than average, to the point that their succession becomes pathological. However, where the description doesn't fit at first glance has to do with the so-called manic phase of what until the nineties was called manic depressive psychosis. The manic state is when people strip naked on the street, or suddenly buy three Ferraris, or feverishly explain to anyone who wants to hear it that what they've got to do is eat guavas, lots and lots of guavas, to save humanity from a third world war. I knew a young guy who did things like that and who, once the crisis had passed, was appalled by what he'd done. He committed suicide, as it seems 20 percent of bipolars do—a more reliable statistic, I'm afraid, than that of Chögyam Trungpa on the amount of time the brain spends focused on the present. I felt sorry for this brilliant, desperate young guy, and never thought I suffered from the same disorder as he did. I was depressive, yes. As I acknowledged honestly in filling out the Vipassana questionnaire, in addition to what can be called empty periods, I've been through two phases of real, severe depression, the sort that lasts several months and during which you hardly ever get up, you can no longer accomplish the most basic tasks, and above all you can no longer imagine that things will change. That's the hallmark of depression: you can't believe that one day you'll get better. Well-meaning friends say, "You'll be fine, you'll see." But you only look at them with dismay and even start to resent them: they're so wide of the mark . . . it's so clear they haven't got a clue . . . When you're in a depression you think that you'll never come out of it, that you won't come out alive, that the only way out is suicide. If you don't commit suicide, however, sooner or later you will come out of it, and then once you're out of it you cross over into the camp of the well-meaning friends and can no longer imagine this state of intolerable and seemingly endless distress. When I was young, I had a bad trip on hallucinogenic mushrooms. They sent me to hell, whose very definition is to be frightful and never-ending. But I was lucid in my nightmare, and told myself: "Don't panic. I took poison. Its effect will last as long as it takes me to digest it, in eight or ten hours it'll be over, I just have to hold on until then." I said this to reassure myself, it was reasonable and true, but at the same time I wondered, "Can I hold on until then? In eight or ten hours *will I still be alive*?" I lived through it, and I know that once you're back among the living you put this hell in perspective, you quickly forget the horror, and that's what I would like not to do in these pages. As Louis-Ferdinand Céline puts it in *Journey to the End of the Night*, "The biggest defeat in every department of life is to forget, especially the things that have done you in." Anyway. Unfortunately for me, I'm no stranger to depression. But what I still didn't know during my first psychiatric consultations is that in the definition of bipolar disorder, the pole opposite the dive into depression isn't necessarily a state of spectacular euphoria and disinhibition that leads to social suicide and often to suicide itself, but just as frequently what psychiatrists call hypomania, which means in plain language that you act like a fool, but not to the same extent. You don't strip naked in the street, you're just at the mercy of the tachypsychia whose name I recently learned. You're bipolar type 2: agitated without necessarily being euphoric, but sometimes also seductive, flirtatious, very sexual, outwardly very much alive, but inclined to make the types of decisions you regret the most while being dead sure that they're right and that you'll never go back on them. Then after that you're dead sure of the very opposite, you realize that you've done the worst thing possible, you try to fix it and do something even worse. You think one thing and then its opposite, you do one thing and then its opposite, in frightening succession. But the worst is that if you're like me and are used to analyzing yourself, once the diagnosis has been reached and the mood swings identified, you gain hindsight, only this hindsight is of little use. Or if it is, it's just to see that no matter what you think, say, or do, you can't trust yourself because there are two of you in the same person, and those two are enemies.

Yoga for Bipolars

The thoughts come thick and fast, twist like flames, burn themselves out, and ignite all over again. One flashes to mind and gives me a thrill. If I can't be cured of this disease, I can describe it. That's my trade. That's what's always

saved me, despite everything. What a great idea! I'll tell
the story of my life from that angle, I'll even reread my
books from that angle, not as literary works but as clinical
documents. The first one that was readable, *The Mustache*,
tells the story of a guy who shaves off his mustache without anyone close to him noticing, not even his wife. At
first he's baffled, then his bafflement spreads and spreads,
turning his life into a nightmare. Is his wife trying to drive
him mad? Is he going mad? Neither of the two hypotheses
is tenable and yet there's no number three, so he goes from
the first to the second and from the second to the first in
a panic-stricken, frightening, tachypsychic oscillation that
leaves him no alternative but escape and, finally, suicide. As
for my last book, *The Kingdom*, its hero is the apostle Paul,
and I now pull out all the stops to cast him as the patron
saint of bipolars, first because his conversion made him not
only the opposite of what he was, but also what he dreaded
to become the most, and second because he spent the rest
of his life in panic-stricken fear of retracing his steps in
the opposite direction. At first glance, my new psychiatric
autobiography project and my upbeat, subtle little book on
yoga—which clearly now belongs to bygone times—have
nothing in common. Nothing at all, except for the fact that
it's both a rule for me and one of the most reliable teachings of psychoanalysis that when you say two things have
nothing in common there are strong chances that on the
contrary they have everything in common, and I remember
very precisely that evening in September 2016 when, sitting alone—as I did almost every evening—on the terrace
of the café Le Rallye, on the corner of Rue de Paradis and

Rue du Faubourg Poissonnière, where I'd just moved, I was blinded like Paul on the road to Damascus by the obvious fact that my psychiatric autobiography and my essay on yoga were in fact *the same book*. Because this illness I suffer from is the deranged, parodic, gruesome version of the great law of alternation whose harmony I so sincerely praised some fifty pages back. From yin is born yang, from yang yin, and you recognize the sage by the fact that he lets himself be wafted gently by the current between the two poles. How do you recognize the madman? By the fact that instead of being wafted by the current he's swept away by it, buffeted from one pole to the other while struggling to keep his head above water, and by the fact that for him yin and yang are not complementary but enemies, both set on his destruction. Everything I was getting ready to say with the calm tone of one who's confidently progressing toward the state of wonder and serenity I see today in a harsh, grim light, the pale light of a dawn execution that I can't help believe is true, truer than the daylight that chases bad dreams away. But I still have one way—just one—to resist the vritti, which is to relate the story of the long and unequal combat I've waged against them all my life. To relate the various attempts I've made all my life to calm the vritti and become what I so desired to be. I love this sentence by the anonymous fourteenth-century English mystic who wrote *The Cloud of Unknowing*: "It is not what you are nor what you have been that God looks at with his merciful eyes, but what you desire to be." What did I desire to be? A stable man, a serene man, a man who could be trusted, a good man, a loving man. Because, of

course, the real thing, and even the only thing, that is at
stake in this combat, the only thing at stake in life, is love,
the ability to love. Disabled as I am, I've tried to bolster
this ability with disciplines like the martial arts, which
aim to foster something inside you other than your ego.
Thirty-five years of writing, thirty years of tai chi, yoga,
and meditation to foster whatever love there is in me: no
one will be able to say I haven't tried, no one will be able to
say I was lazy, no one will be able to say I didn't fight. "Give
up, my heart," writes Michaux, "we have battled enough.
And let my life stop. We've not been cowards, we've done
what we could." Yes, we've done what we could, and you
can't say the long and unequal combat did much good. At
the same time, I'm aware that such thoughts are thoughts
of the night, thoughts of madness and sickness, and that
they're not what I always think. At other times in my life, I
believed I was this stable, loving man, this man who could
be trusted. And neither I nor the women who loved me
were mistaken in believing it. This life, my poor, miserable,
sometimes vibrant, sometimes loving life, has not been all
delusion and defeat and madness, and the cardinal sin is
to forget that. In the darkness, it's crucial to remember that
you've also lived in the light, and that the light is no less
true than the darkness. And I'm certain my book can be a
good book, a necessary book, if it can hold these two poles
together: on the one hand a long aspiration for unity, for
light, for empathy, and on the other the powerful, oppos-
ing force of division, self-immurement, and despair. This
tension is more or less what everyone has to deal with,

only with me it takes on an extreme, pathological form. But since I'm a writer I can do something with it. I must do something with it. My own sad story can take on a universal character: that's what I say to myself, sitting on the terrace of Le Rallye, and I remember I even asked the waitress, a smart young Chinese girl with whom I chatted from time to time, if she thought that *Yoga for Bipolars* was a good title for a book. The question puzzled her, but to be on the safe side and to make me happy, she said she thought it was.

"And in the morning, the wolf a-a-ate her"

To boost my confidence, I repeat to myself that if I can work seriously on this story, I'll be able to wrest an hour or two a day from the vritti. A form of meditation, a combat as heroic as that of Monsieur Seguin's goat in the story by Alphonse Daudet. I've often identified with that daring, hapless nanny goat who wanted to see what the world was like beyond the fences, and who ran through the forests, over the hills, drunk with freedom and disdain for her timid companions who stayed in the enclosure. She paid for it dearly, as you probably know. Stalked by the wolf, she struggled and struggled all night to escape. When I was young I had a record on which the actor Fernandel told Daudet's tale, and his southern accent, normally so good-natured and comical, made the last sentence sound incredibly threatening: "And in the morning, the wolf a-a-ate her."

I can still hear this sentence just as he said it, it scares me as much now as it did when I was six, and I'm afraid that as I approach sixty that's just what awaits me: that the wolf will e-e-eat me, too, and that I'll never make it back to the warmth of the enclosure.

The Gemini twins separated

It was totally predictable, since manic excitement is followed invariably by a dive into depression. An atrocious
period. In the first phase I was elated at the prospect
of a new book and a new life, full of promises and con-
quests. I rented quite a nice apartment on Rue du Faubourg Poissonnière. I bought a Bluetooth speaker and took
out a subscription to Deezer, both of which I imagined,
oddly enough, as attributes of my new life—modest attributes, to be sure, and a far cry from buying Ferraris on a
whim. Then I end up as lonely as a rat, without a woman,
or impotent when by chance I bring one home, my neck
covered in dandruff, my cock blistered with herpes, unable
to write, having lost all faith in this book project that a few
weeks earlier seemed so right, so necessary, so doable, as
all I had to do was start by describing what was happening

to me. The problem is that I don't know what's happening to me, and I'm no longer able to tell myself or anyone else anything at all. To live you need a story, and I no longer have one. My life is reduced to the path between my bed, where I bathe in a terrible sweat, and the terrace of the café Le Rallye, where I spend hours smoking cigarette after cigarette in a dazed stupor, under the worried eye of the nice Chinese waitress who to please me had told me she liked the title *Yoga for Bipolars*. Even today I can't walk past this café without a shudder. For almost two months I barely washed or changed my clothes. The bathtub got clogged and I did nothing to fix it, and even when I went to bed I barely changed out of my depressed man's garb: shapeless corduroy pants, an old sweater full of holes, sneakers whose laces I'd removed as if in anticipation of the precautions that would soon be imposed on me in the psychiatric hospital. I don't stop trembling, objects fall from my hands. If I put jars of yogurt in the fridge, they slip and crash onto the kitchen floor. Yogurt I can deal with, but one day I wanted to move the little Gemini statue, which I'd placed on a shelf like an altar, by a few inches, and I dropped that, too. It shattered. I stood there for at least an hour, looking at these pieces of terra-cotta that had been the secret symbol of my love, between my feet on the parquet floor, and I thought, there you go, you couldn't say it more eloquently, everything was broken, nothing could be repaired, it was all over.

Wyatt Mason's article

It was around this time that an American journalist and writer named Wyatt Mason came to meet me to write a long portrait for *The New York Times Magazine*. At any other time this visit and the interest of *The New York Times Magazine* would have pleased me no end, because for a long time now I've aspired to a higher profile in the Anglophone literary world. But at this moment I couldn't care less about my profile in the Anglophone literary world, I'm totally incapable of being pleased about anything, and that's what jumps out at Wyatt Mason as soon as I open the door to my apartment on Rue du Faubourg Poissonnière. It's an objectively pleasant duplex apartment with large windows facing a leafy courtyard, he notes at the beginning of his article. Except that like its tenant, this empty apartment in which there wasn't the least trace of life—no books, no pictures, no chosen anything—had a strangely grim-cheerful, vaguely creepy air of vacancy. It's rare for journalists to write such intimate impressions of the person they interview. It's the kind of thing I could do, and Wyatt Mason did it with kind, apologetic delicacy. I remember him well: a guy in his forties with a shaved head, short beard, soft voice, very friendly, whom I'm happy to call to the witness stand to give an account of this period of my life I otherwise recall so badly. His article, which I've just found on the website of *The New York Times*, starts as follows:

> Late last October, as American electoral pandemonium was approaching its climax, I was in a living

room in Paris where the 59-year-old French writer
Emmanuel Carrère was talking about shame. Carrère, who has the silhouette of someone half his age
but whose face is so deeply grooved that its lines
seem carved there, wasn't speaking abstractly.

More or less at the same time, another American journalist described me as rather handsome despite having a
slightly simian face with protruding, bat-like ears and close-
set eyes like those of George W. Bush. But to come back to
Wyatt Mason, whom I receive reclining like an analysand
on a black leather couch that, he writes with a talent that
strikes me on rereading his article today, "seemed somehow
forlorn, abandoned, a huge dog of a couch waiting miserably for its owner to return." One thing that Wyatt Mason
doesn't know, and which he'd certainly have been able to
make good use of, is that two years earlier the haggard,
trembling man in front of him was photographed on this
same couch in a lotus pose with a smiling, serene look on
his face, and that this photo adorned the cover of a weekly
that opened its dossier on meditation with a long interview
with him. And yes, I talk about shame. The first thing I tell
in this context is a story about General Massu, a French
general of the highest rank during the Algerian War. That
was a dirty war—to the extent that any war can be dirty or
clean, that is—made up of fierce skirmishes, nocturnal
disappearances, civilians slaughtered like sheep, and inter-
rogations that took place, on the French side, using two
main techniques: the bathtub and the *gégène*. The gégène,
as I explain to Wyatt Mason, and as he in turn explains to

his readers, involves torture with electric prods from a generator, applied to the temples, ears, and, if the person being interrogated is a man, to his balls. Later, in the early
seventies, General Massu was accused of having tortured
many people. Without denying it, he justified this practice
by saying that you have to choose the lesser of two evils,
and that if that's what it takes to save dozens of lives, such
extreme solutions are necessary. That's what torturers often say, but Massu, in an interview with the same weekly
that would photograph me on my couch in a sage's outfit
fifty years later, then went off on another tangent. "Listen.
Don't exaggerate. The prods? I tried them on myself. It
hurts, but not worse than that." I repeat this sentence to
Wyatt Mason: "*I tried them on myself,*" inviting him to appreciate this fascinating blend of bullshit and obscenity.
Because someone who applies prods to himself can stop
anytime he wants, when it starts to really hurt. But what's
atrocious about torture is that someone else is doing it to
you, and you don't know when he'll stop. Why am I saying
all this? Wyatt Mason understands very well. And he explains very well to his readers that someone like me, who
doesn't write fiction but autobiographical texts whose first
rule is not to lie, someone for whom literature is above all
else *the place where you don't lie,* is in two very different
moral situations depending on whether he's talking about
himself or about other people. I've been told from time to
time that it takes a lot of guts to paint yourself in an unflat-
tering light the way I do in my books. That's not true, I tell
Wyatt Mason. It's not courage, or if it's courage it's the
same kind of courage General Massu displays when he

uses the generator on himself. Like him, I can stop when I want, I can say what I want and not say what I want, I'm the one with my finger on the button. But when you write about others you switch—or can switch—over to real torture, because the person who's writing has full power and the person he's writing about is at his mercy. Ten years ago, I also say to Wyatt Mason—who knows perfectly what I'm talking about, his professionalism amazes me—I published an autobiographical book called *My Life as a Russian Novel*. I laid myself bare in that book, fine, that's my business, but I also subjected two other people to the same treatment: my mother, who was afraid I'd reveal a family secret, and my companion at the time, about whose emotional and sexual life I revealed details on the pretext that, as they were inextricably intertwined with my own, they were as much a part of my life as they were of hers. This twofold unpackaging produced suffering but no catastrophes, thank goodness. Still: I crossed a line that shouldn't have been crossed. My next book, *Lives Other Than My Own*, told intimate details about several people, but I had them read the manuscript before it was published and they okayed it, so that book, which deals with sad and even terrible events, was written with serenity, and remains by far my favorite work because it gave me the illusion, shared by many readers, that I was a good man. But it, too, is an illusion, I tell Wyatt Mason. I am not a good man. I'd like to be one, I'd give my body and soul to be one, because I'm an eminently moral individual who distinguishes very clearly between good and evil and places nothing higher than goodness,

but alas, no, I'm not good, and I quote to Wyatt Mason—
how many times have I quoted it, how many times have I
repeated it to myself—the question Saint Paul puts to
God, no doubt the only being to whom you can ask such a
thing: "Why do I not do the good that I love but the evil
that I hate?" It's clear that at this point Wyatt Mason no
longer sees what I'm saying as the reflections of a responsi-
ble man, but as symptoms of an alarming state of distress
for which he shows true compassion. "Carrère," he wrote,
"who is nothing if not exquisitely polite and who tries at
every turn to express himself with precision and care and
frankness and good cheer, did his best to be a good host,
offering tea, offering himself as much as he could. But in
retrospect, he was, in fact, suffering terribly." So ends the
first part of his article and the first day we spent together,
because it was a long portrait, eight pages of *The New York
Times Magazine*, Wyatt Mason had come to Paris specially
for that, and it had been agreed that the interview would
cover two days. What to do with the second? Having ex-
hausted the charms of the monologue on the couch that
resembled a forlorn dog, the idea was to break out of the
static, conventional format of the interview in favor of
something a little livelier. To do something I liked to do, for
example, go somewhere I liked to go: a street market, a
good restaurant, a soccer game . . . When Wyatt Mason
asked me if I had any ideas, I took him to the terrace of Le
Rallye, hoping he'd be satisfied with the cliché of the typical Parisian café where the writer comes every morning to
have his double espresso and croissant, observe the other

customers, and ideally jot down notes in a small notebook. The idea might have been good, but I overdid it. When the Chinese waitress came to take our order, I overplayed my status as a regular with a stridently exuberant greeting, which she received as if I'd gone mad. Wyatt Mason drank his coffee thoughtfully, then asked if I liked Rembrandt. I think that not many people will answer no to that question, but the fact is that yes, I love Rembrandt. The guy spent his whole life anxiously scrutinizing his own face: how could he not be my favorite painter, even? So Wyatt Mason suggested we go to see an exhibition of Rembrandt prints that had just opened at the Jacquemart-André Museum. I said okay. It was certainly better than going to some fancy restaurant where I couldn't swallow a thing, not even an appetizer, or an "amuse-bouche" as they say; and I don't know why I suggested that instead of taking a taxi we could go there on my scooter. This scooter ride, more than the Rembrandt exhibit, about which there wasn't much to say, is the high point of Wyatt Mason's article. He's not the only passenger to describe my driving style as careful, perhaps a little too careful, even, in fact so careful it's dangerous, with a tremendous amount of unexpected braking, and turns taken so slowly that the scooter risks tipping over and falling under its own weight. Jolted and tossed in this way, increasingly tense behind me, Wyatt Mason describes the sound made by the front of his helmet hitting the back of mine each time I brake, the effort he puts into preventing the front of his helmet from hitting the back of mine, and that's where he writes this amazing thing that even more than all the rest inspires in me such profound sympathy:

> This would be a lot easier if we were close friends, brothers, and it were natural to rest against him. Of course, I didn't do this, because it would have been awkward for an American reporter to embrace his just-met subject on the back of a scooter. But the feeling that seized me, and it was oddly powerful, was that I should. That everything would be a lot better if I did, if I just reached out and held on.

The walled-up little boy

Wyatt Mason's article doesn't end with this passage, which is so remarkable for its literary and human qualities, but with these lines: "However preoccupied Carrère is with loss and violence and pain, his books move to endings that earn a space of joy. They are written by someone who knows precisely what they cost." It's strange to read this sentence today, as I make my way toward the end of this book and try to create a space of joy there. I'm searching, groping. I don't yet know what form it may take, but I think it's possible. Joy, or at least its possibility, has returned to my life. Love, or at least its possibility, has returned to my life. If someone had said that to me three and a half years ago when I was living on Rue du Faubourg Poissonnière, I wouldn't have believed it. I'd even have found such a prediction insulting because it was so misplaced. I was sure that my sadness would last forever, and that if I still managed to write anything, as I believed less and less, it would be to say exactly that: that this sadness would last forever, that I'd remain walled up in it forever. Some twenty years ago, while reading the newspaper *Libération*, I came across a news item that marked me for life. The parents of a four-year-old boy had taken him to the hospital for a minor operation. He was due to get out the next day. But the anesthesiologist made a mistake, and despite weeks of desperate care, the little boy remained deaf, dumb, blind, and paralyzed. Irreversibly, for good. When I read that, I was shaken to the core. Nothing has ever upset me as much as that. I couldn't think of anything else. I couldn't think of anything but the moment when the little boy wakes up. The moment he regains consciousness, in the dark. Worried at first, but the way you worry when you know your worries will end. His parents can't be far away. They'll turn on the light, talk to him. But nothing comes. No light. No sound. He tries to move, but he can't. To scream, but he can't hear himself. Maybe he can feel someone touching him, opening his mouth to feed him. Maybe he's fed intravenously, the article doesn't say. His parents and the hospital staff stand around his bed, speechless with horror, but he doesn't know. It's impossible to communicate with him, impossible to reach him. He's not in a coma. They know that he's conscious, that behind his pinched, waxy face, behind his unseeing gaze, a living, walled-up little boy is silently screaming in horror. No one can explain the situation to him, and who'd have the courage? No one can imagine what's going on in his mind, how he makes sense of what's happening to him. There are no words for it. I have no words. I who am otherwise so articulate have no way of expressing what this appalling story awakens in me. Something deep inside me, something that lies at the root of my own experience, that constitutes the reality of reality, the bottom line, the last word. And it's not the space of inalienable joy toward which Wyatt Mason sees my books evolving, but the absolute horror, the unspeakable terror of a four-year-old boy who regains consciousness in eternal darkness.

François Roustang's last advice

One day, nonetheless, I did leave my apartment on the corner of Rue du Faubourg Poissonnière and Rue du Paradis to see the old psychoanalyst François Roustang in his dark mezzanine office on Rue de Naples. This extraordinary man who had been a Jesuit, then a disciple of Lacan, had escaped from these two churches at the end of his long life to become a sort of Zen master. He had quite the physical presence, with a polished head, pale blue eyes, and impassive features: I've never met anyone who was so tangibly rooted in the center of gravity that the Japanese locate in the pit of the stomach and call the *hara*. I've visited him three times at crucial moments in my life, and his words have always been both brutal and illuminating. The last time had been ten years ago, in the second of my three major depressions. At length I explained to him that life had brought me to a dead end from which there was no exit, and that the only way out for me was suicide. When you say something like that, you expect to be contradicted. But instead of contradicting me, Roustang had said softly: "You're right. Suicide doesn't get very good press these days, but sometimes it's the right solution." I looked at him, stunned. If there's one thing a therapist of any persuasion cannot say, it's that suicide is the right solution. Then he added, "Or you can live." You can understand why I say that he was something of a Zen master. It was as if this sentence—"Or you can live"—resulted in a psychic short circuit that allowed me not only to get out of my depression, but also to live a full and happy life for the next ten years. And now, ten years later, here I was at his office once again, just as convinced that I'd never find a way out of my depression, that I was doomed to shame and horror, that there was nothing left but suicide. He let me go on like that for a while, then this time he cut me off in midsentence. "Shut up now." What could I do? I stopped talking. So did he. We were silent, for maybe five minutes. Five minutes is a very long time. He looked at me calmly, without looking away, almost without blinking, but without excessive intensity. Under his gaze, I remembered something Albert Speer, the architect of the Third Reich, relates in his memoirs, and which I haven't read anywhere else: very often, in the most varied circumstances, Hitler indulged in the childish game of staring people down. It was a duel, a cruel and dangerous duel that he always won, of course, because no one dared to challenge him, but which you couldn't lose too quickly either, for fear of cutting short his pleasure. The way Roustang plunged his blue eyes into mine, his dense, inert calm, was the exact opposite: no challenge, no conflict, no tension, no competition. I could feel deep waves of stillness emanating from him, like the voice of S. N. Goenka. Finally, he said: "What you're going through is horrible: fine. Live it. Embrace it. Be nothing more than this horror. If you must die, die. Don't look for a reason or a way out. Do nothing, let go: that's the only way things can change." In other words: meditate, because meditation is exactly that.

The Blood Quran

I tried to obey Roustang, that is, to do nothing, but it didn't work. So I tried to do something else: a news report. I've always enjoyed this sort of work, sometimes it's saved me: dressing up as Alex Térieur and going out into the field. Summoning what little energy I had, I called my friend and editor-in-chief Patrick de Saint-Exupéry. Patrick heads the magazine *XXI*, and I call him my editor-in-chief even though I don't work exclusively for *XXI* or any other publication because when I have an idea for a story I suggest it to him, and because he sometimes suggests, to me, stories that have always turned out to be excellent. I tell him that I'm going through a tough time—"Judging from your voice," he told me later, "it was a *really* tough time"—and that it would be good for me to get a change of air. It speaks both for his imagination and for his friendship that he called me back a week later to suggest the following story. In 1999, Saddam Hussein's eldest son, Uday, a dangerous psycho-

path, escaped an assassination attempt. To thank Allah, his
father made the strange vow to have a Quran written with
his own blood. For two years, a nurse came to the presi-
dential palace each week to take Saddam's blood, which
she then took to Iraq's most famous calligrapher. Once
finished, the Blood Quran was displayed with great pomp
in a mosque built by Saddam, known at the time as the
"Mother of All Battles Mosque," which is remarkable for
this architectural singularity: its minarets are in the shape
of Kalashnikovs. Then the Americans arrived, the already
chaotic country was plunged even deeper into chaos—a bit
like how I will soon go from "significant moral suffering"
to "intense moral suffering"—and the Blood Quran disappeared. No one knows where it is now, few people actually
care, but Patrick thought first of all that a story about it
would be a good introduction to today's Iraq, and second—
and above all—that this adventurous and even dangerous
trip, this adrenaline shot, was the best thing he could do
for a friend who was losing his grip. There really are people you can count on in life. I like the idea. And I like it
all the more because with a bit of luck I could get killed
in a car bombing, and it seems to me that going to Baghdad will be less of a feat than crossing Rue du Faubourg
Poissonnière. The problem is that you don't go to Baghdad
just like that, it takes time to get the visas. I say the *visas*
because Patrick has the idea of sending two of us: me, who
knows nothing about Iraq, and Lucas Menget, a seasoned
international reporter who knows it like the back of his
hand. Lucas and I got on excellently when we finally went
there almost a year later. In the meantime, our story con-

sists of weekly or even biweekly visits to the Iraqi consulate
to inquire into the status of our visas. These visits were
my only outings that winter, and strangely enough I have
quite fond memories of them. I'd get off at the Porte Dau-
phine station and slowly walk up the snowy, supernaturally
wide Avenue Foch, where luxurious black sedans passed
by silently as if in slow motion, toward the consulate. Our
appointments were with a mustached diplomat—all Iraqis
have mustaches—who would seat us ceremoniously on a
deep, hideous sofa before sitting down opposite us on an
equally deep, hideous sofa, separated by a canyon of four or
five yards, and who, once we were settled, would have little tulip-shaped glasses brought in to us with a very strong,
very sweet tea that I found more and more delicious with
every passing visit. Lucas and the diplomat knew each
other well and had many acquaintances in common, and
would proceed to exchange news about them and their
families. These conversations, full of political innuendo
that was completely lost on me, were all part of the obstacle course aimed at getting a visa, but both Lucas and the
diplomat seemed to enjoy them, and I ended up enjoying
them too. I wasn't asked to participate, so I took little sips
of my delicious tea on the hideous sofa, the hours passed
unhurriedly in these offices where no one seemed rushed,
the small talk went on and on, and it was also due to the
presence of Lucas, who is incredibly calm, decent, and reassuring, really a solid gold guy, that I felt safe. Yes: during
this atrocious winter, the only place I felt safe was in the
Iraqi consulate.

The patient on admission

My internment at the Sainte-Anne Psychiatric Hospital lasted four months. The medical report, which I have in front of me, begins with this summary: "Characteristic depressive episode with melancholic elements and suicidal ideas in the context of a type 2 bipolar disorder." And, a little further on, here's how the patient is described on admission:

> Moderate psychomotor retardation with hypomimia, sad expression but emotional reactivity. Despondency, anhedonia, abulia, significant moral suffering, asthenia with a considerable psychic and physical toll incurred in carrying out daily activities. Melancholic elements with pejoration of the future and a sense of incurability. Ruminations, feelings of guilt toward loved ones, invasive suicidal ideations . . .

You don't have to master psychiatric vocabulary to understand that I wasn't doing well. If you want to go into the
nuances, "significant moral suffering" is worrying, but less
so than "intense moral suffering," which I was soon to experience, and which is itself less worrying than "intolerable
moral suffering." I've experienced that, too, I don't know if
there's a fourth. In the past few days, my already not very
glorious state has worsened. Our visas for Iraq have eluded
us week after week, and with them my dreams of an adventurous escape or—hardly less desirable—death in a car
bombing. From one day to the next, from one hour to the
next, I was first tachypsychic then catatonic, and this state
so alarmed my sister Nathalie that she made an appoint-
ment for me at Sainte-Anne. That's how we ended up on
the top floor of a modern building on the edge of the hospital compound, in front of a cordial sixty-year-old man in
a white coat, with bright blue eyes and the quiet authority
that characterizes what's known as a bigwig—even though
no one ever talks of anyone being a little wig—who, seeing
me in the state described in the report, decides to admit
me straight off. I don't go home, they put me to bed, we'll
have to wait and see for how long. As for Iraq, which I
brought up at the start of the consultation, the big shot
is sorry but it'll have to wait, there'll still be time for that
in a few months. He stresses the notion of illness—very
different from that of neurosis, which has dominated my
adult life. The question is not to discover its origin or to
understand why I've spent my life lugging such a big load
of shit around in my head. The fact is that I'm sick, just

as sick as if I'd had a stroke or peritonitis, so they're going
to lay me down and look for the right treatment, and they
don't hide the fact that they're groping in the dark and that
they might not find just the right thing for me right away.
"But what we can do until we find it," says the bigwig, "is
keep you out of harm's way. And don't worry, we'll get you
out of here as fast as we can." Hearing this, I heave a sigh
of relief: I'm sick, I'm going to lie down, stop fighting, let
things take their course, they'll take care of me, and for
starters they'll shoot me up big-time.

The protocol

To return to the medical report: "Inclusion in a protocol
with twice-weekly administration of ketamine. First three
infusions: good tolerance, thymic improvement." Ketamine,
for those who don't know, is a horse anesthetic that teenagers use to get high, and which in recent years has been
found to have antidepressant properties. This is my introduction to high psychiatric chemistry. Before and after
each session, the protocol includes my being given a questionnaire, which is no longer about my meditation experience, as in the happy days when I thought I was on my
way to a state of wonder and serenity, but about my desire
to live or to die, my suicidal impulses, my "pejoration of
the future," et cetera. First infusion: forty minutes, not one
more or less, and when it's over, it's over, from one moment
to the next. But during these forty minutes it's an XXL
high. Lying in bed, I remain conscious, perfectly conscious.

I can feel time passing. I can hear the doctor and the nurse talking softly. But I get the impression that they're far, far below me, lost in the landscape above which I'm floating. Because I am floating. I'm drifting. I see everything. I'm perfectly calm, perfectly fine, I'd like it to last forever. It's like the descriptions of near-death experiences, and of heroin, of course. The heroin that you should never touch because it's *so good*. I'm glad I'm interned at Sainte-Anne if they're going to drug me so wonderfully. I feel good. Even after the first three infusions I feel good, my tolerance to the drug is so encouraging, my thymic improvement so obvious that I'm already talking about leaving, and not just about leaving the hospital but about leaving the country. With ketamine, Iraq is back on the agenda. I even ask the doctors about the possibility of taking a few doses to Baghdad and having them administered by a local nurse, why not the one—ha ha!—who took Saddam's blood? Calm down, they say patiently, calm down.

"Your brother has requested euthanasia. What do we do?"

"Fourth injection: bad tolerance with intense moral suffering and request for euthanasia." Intense moral suffering and request for euthanasia: things take a turn for the worse, we're into the rough. Even though I was full of confidence before this fourth injection. A few more and, seeing how things got off to such a good start, I already saw myself in the clear. Then, the night before the infusion, I freak out. Although I've forgotten so much, I remember very well that my anxiety had its starting point in one of the most perfidious aspects of bipolar disorder. When you're in the depressive phase, there's no getting around the fact that you're there: it's horrible, it's hell, but at least you can't be wrong about it. What's insidious about the manic phase is that you don't realize it's a manic phase. Especially when it's only hypomanic and you're not stripping down in the street or buying a Ferrari. You tell yourself that you're fine, that everything's all right. After all, that can happen: it's normal, desirable even. You know it won't last forever, but when it happens you have every reason to be happy and not to tell yourself that it's a trap. In my case, however, there's a good chance that it is a trap, another blow that the disease has in store for me. Because it's no longer me but the disease that wields power over me. The disease lies to me, the disease deceives me. The more I believe I'm doing fine, mastering my life, riding the wave, the more I deceive myself and prepare for the depressive dive that follows these periods of well-being and confidence. And worst of all is when I'm in love. For everyone, being in love is a sort of manic phase, the most desirable of manic phases. But I, and unfortunate people like me, have no right to desire these manic phases. I have no right to trust them, and if I'm honest I have to warn any woman who enters my life not to trust them either. She must know that the wonderful man she's fallen in love with—because I can be wonderful, believe me—can turn into a catatonic depressive or, worse still, an enemy, from one minute to the next. If I don't want to cause suffering, love is now forbidden to me.

No more love. No more enchantment of being in love, the best thing in the world. No more believing—no, forget believing: *being sure*—that this one is the one you've been waiting for all your life without knowing it, and who was waiting for you, too. No more going down to buy a fresh baguette and squeezing oranges before she wakes up. No more following her with your eyes when she walks around the apartment wearing only your T-shirt. No more texting thirty times a day, loving her words and knowing she loves yours, no more her sending you a picture of her breasts in the mirror when she's in a fitting room, which makes you want to stand behind her and cup them in your palms and feel their weight in your hands. No more seeing the look on her face when you enter her, and no more sighing "Oh" at the same moment because it's so good. Life may go on, but what's it worth without all of that? As I slide down this slope, the night is atrocious. I hear bloodcurdling screams that can't be real, and must resound only in my sick brain. In the morning, all I want is the ketamine shot that will send me to heaven for at least half an hour. I want it so much that, fearing I won't be given it if I confess to my psychological state, I say in the questionnaire that I didn't sleep well and that I had some dark thoughts but that in fact I'm fine. The drip begins. I welcome with gratitude the blissful liquefaction that morphine, heroin, and all the opiates procure, and then very quickly things take a turn for the worse. I'm heading for death. It's clear: I'm heading for death. The doctors murmur softly to the right of my bed, I don't understand what they're saying but they must be reciting verses from the *Tibetan Book of the Dead* to accompany me to the Bardo. There's a light above me. I have to go there. I have to go there. I mustn't miss the exit. I mustn't remain in this in-between state, this bad life. Everything must end and the suffering must stop, for good. Several times I go to the enormous effort—when you're on ketamine, every word costs you dearly—of repeating "I want to die, I want to die." Instead of two doctors there are now four or five in my room, which becomes too small, much too small, a small box that shrinks even more, and, stuck to the ceiling, I start to cry. I cry, I cry, I say that I want to die, that I know very well that it's not their job to kill me, but I beg them to do it anyway. Finally, in response to my moans and my begging that they kill me, or failing that, that they at least turn off my mind, that's what they do, and quickly. One shot, the fuses blow, everyone's gone. Then begins a blank that lasts several days and would end this chapter if I didn't have one more sentence to add. What I'm saying here is brutal, but my condition was brutal and I'd like it to be clear that the doctors I dealt with at Sainte-Anne were and are all very competent, but hey, there are jerks everywhere, and as things turned out there was one who called Nathalie after this episode and asked: "Your brother has requested euthanasia. What do we do?"

The secure unit

After my request for euthanasia I was transferred to the secure unit. How long did I spend there? I would have said three or four days, in fact it was two weeks. That was where the monotonous, haunting screams I'd heard the night before my disastrous fourth infusion, and which I'd thought existed only in my head, came from. In fact, they came from the room right next to where I was now. All the doors in the secure unit have frosted glass panes except for the one to that room, which is fitted with wood or plywood, with the aim, I thought, of protecting the nurses from some kind of Hannibal the Cannibal of whom I never caught a glimpse. I share my room with a young guy who is certainly not dangerous but who has the most distressing symptoms of madness: stupor, a shrill voice, dragging his feet in slippers, drooling, and never changing out of his pajamas. That said, I guess I didn't exactly cut a sterling figure either.

Nathalie found me one day semiconscious in my bed, asking where I was and crooning sadly: "I want to go home,
I want to die at home, take me home . . ." In my hospital
report that translates as: "A brief episode of derealization
followed by frank delirium with spatiotemporal disorienta-
tion, anxiety, and acute feeling of strangeness." Something
like that doesn't fill you with confidence, that's for sure,
but I got through it, they did what they had to for that. I
was able to leave the secure unit, go back up to the third
floor and resume a normal hospital life, made up of long,
lethargic naps, cups of weak hot chocolate in the cafeteria,
reading spells, half-hearted attempts to resume my essay
on yoga, tray meals as quickly defecated as eaten because
even though I was on morphine—which normally consti-
pates you—I was shitting every quarter of an hour, and ca-
sual, passing friendships. My companions in the ward were
an elegant woman with stylish hair who confessed with
melancholic pride that this was her seventeenth long-term
stay, and an obese film critic whom I'd known in a previous
life, lost sight of for thirty years and who was having a good
little depression—well, a good *big* one: you don't end up at
Sainte-Anne otherwise. He used to write for a magazine
that was a direct rival to mine, and we had a good time
talking about the people we knew and our past quarrels.
One day as we were pushing our trays in the cafeteria, a
very young woman came up and started talking to me as if
she knew me well, and we ended up sitting together at the
same table, the film critic, she, and I. The film critic got
all tied in knots, as if I wanted to hit on this twenty-two-

year-old and he was getting in the way. The young woman said placidly that she was completely crazy, but that after a dozen electroshocks—which she called ECTs—she was doing better. She knew me better than I thought, because she'd been in the secure unit at the same time as me, only she remembered it and I didn't. She remembered that we'd talked a lot, especially about Cormac McCarthy's novels, which she loved, as did I apparently—which surprised me, because although I vaguely intend to do so one day, I haven't read any of Cormac McCarthy's novels. Did I pretend to have read them to please her? There was so much familiarity—complicity even—in her attitude that I wondered if there was even more to our friendship than this camaraderie between patients. If so, it never made it past the doors of the secure unit.

The fairy garden

This very slight improvement didn't last, and was soon followed by "feelings of distress and incurability, numerous bouts of tears, invasive suicidal thoughts involving a hanging scenario without any immediate plans to follow through." I can tell you a little more about this "hanging scenario without any immediate plans to follow through," and especially about the setting. One afternoon I'm walking in this city within a city that is the hospital compound. I don't know if you can call such atrocious rambling *walking*, nevertheless by putting one foot in front of the other I wind up in an area where the alleyways all bear the names of artists afflicted with mental illness: Maurice Utrillo, Vincent Van Gogh, Maurice Ravel. They're kidding, I think to myself, why Ravel? He was neurotic, but not crazy. I walk from the alleyways to the covered galleries between the wards, and at one point I see a door that opens onto a large deserted garden enclosed by what seem like disused brick buildings. An empty, silent enclave, without patients or doctors, untended, strewn with dead leaves, planted with chestnut trees with black trunks and pruned branches. The pallid, psychiatric version of "The Fairy Garden," the last piece of Ravel's *Mother Goose* suite, which is indeed fairylike. The ideal place to carry out my project. The lowest branches are more than two yards above the ground, and there's a pile of rusty garden chairs along one wall. All I need to do is climb up on one of them and kick it away. My feet will twitch ten or so inches above the ground. It's not much, but it's enough: you're just as dead ten inches above the ground as you are two yards up, the same way you're just as drowned five inches underwater as you are ten yards down. All that's missing is a rope and the right moment to do it without being discovered. I nurtured this little scenario for a few days, and even found an old hardware shop that sold clothesline, not far from the hospital on Rue de la Gaîté. Then I went back to the corner of Allée Maurice Ravel and didn't see the open door again. It wasn't just that it wasn't open anymore: it was no longer there. I searched and searched, in vain. Maybe that door never existed.

The lost room

I once read a fascinating little book by Roger Caillois called *The Uncertainty That Comes from Dreams*. In it he tells a story that has never stopped haunting me. The dreamer is a man walking in the Ternes neighborhood in Paris. He knows where he's going, he's happy to be going there. From the metro station where he's just got off the train, he's familiar with the route. He could walk it with his eyes closed, describe it down to the last detail. And if he likes taking it so much, it's because it leads him to the street and the building where a woman with whom he's had an absolutely secret affair for more than ten years lives. This affair is the most precious thing in the world to him. Once every two weeks—they've agreed on this schedule—he gets off at the Ternes metro and walks for five minutes to the quiet little street and fashionable building where the woman's apartment is located. She opens the door, they embrace, the door closes behind them, and the hours that follow are theirs alone. In this bubble of space and time, totally sheltered from the outside world, everything is desire, softness, tranquillity, understanding between bodies, murmured conversation. They both know that nothing like this would be possible if they lived together, as they've sometimes thought of doing. It's in secrecy that their love unfolds, and they both believe that, protected in this way, it will last forever. Until one of them dies, they'll meet once every two weeks in the peace of this flat toward which the man is confidently heading. On he walks, along the avenue leading to the street of his happiness. But he must not have been paying attention, he's passed the street, that's never happened to him before. He walks back up the avenue. And he doesn't find the street. There's the street above it, the street below it, both of which he knows perfectly well, but the street he's looking for, which should be between the two, is no longer there. He walks up and down several times, as if he were waiting for the street to return to its place, but it's not there anymore. This isn't possible, the man thinks, I know the route by heart, from the station to the avenue, the avenue to the street, the street to the building, the building to the apartment. But as soon as he thinks this, he realizes that in fact he doesn't remember a thing: not the street that's just disappeared, or the building, or the apartment, whose floor plan he could have drawn from memory and which has now been swallowed up by oblivion, not even the face of the woman who was secretly the great love of his life. He no longer remembers her face, he no longer remembers her voice, he no longer remembers the words she said to him, he no longer remembers her name. None of this exists anymore, because none of it, he understands, ever existed. This marvelous woman, this enchanted affair, was nothing but a dream. And it's at this moment, when the man realizes that the most precious thing in his life was only a dream, that he wakes up. And now comes the most poignant part of Roger Caillois's story: all of that was nothing but a dream, a classic dream of anxiety, but the dreamer experiences in real life the same feeling of absolute distress as his double in the dream. This precious possession—the woman, their affair, the shared secret—he owned only in the dream and he lost only in the dream. It happened in a second, but in that second, ten years of mad love unfolded, and what he's left with is their loss. As if this marvelous chunk of the past had really been given to him and had really just been taken away from him, leaving him distressed, bereaved, dizzy with loss. And every time I think of this dream that Roger Caillois either dreamed or invented, as I'm now doing in the cafeteria of the Sainte-Anne Psychiatric Hospital, I also feel distressed, bereaved, and dizzy, making me want not just to die but *to be dead*, to have never existed myself.

"I continue not to die"

My friend Ruth Zylberman sent me these two short letters, from an eight-year-old boy to his grandmother during the 1936 purges in the Soviet Union. The first:

> Dear Babushka, I'm not dead yet. You're the only one I have in the world and I'm the only one you have. If I don't die, when I'm grown up and you're very, very old, I'll work and take care of you. Your grandson, Gavrik.

And the second:

> Dear Babushka, I didn't die this time either. It's not the time I told you about in my last letter. I continue not to die.

The poster for the Dufy exhibition

It's a beach in Normandy or Brittany, at any rate on France's northwest coast. A pier juts out into the waves. The sky is cloudy and luminous. Women in dresses and hats sit on folding chairs or on the sand, watching children play. It's a peaceful, straightforward painting, the poster for an exhibition of works by Raoul Dufy, faded and discolored like the posters that decorate waiting rooms where the magazines aren't renewed either. This beach, this painting, this poster, are for me the saddest sight in the world. Not just the saddest: also the most frightening. I hope I never see them again. Just thinking about them, dreaming about them, is going to the place you must absolutely not go. It's the bad place par excellence, the worst place. This poster, this picture, this beach, are the first thing I saw when I resurfaced in the recovery room after the electroshocks, which are administered under general anesthesia. When I regained consciousness, I was lying on a stretcher. There were other stretchers around me, and other patients on stretchers, but I couldn't see them. It's strange, I think as I write this, that my stretcher was always turned in such a way that when I opened my eyes I always, always, saw that beach and those women in hoop dresses watching their children in sailor suits. It's strange, but that's how it is. I remember each re-awakening as a moment of unbearable distress. What made it unbearable was that it was impossible to consider it as a moment that could be put into perspective and would be followed by better moments. It wasn't a moment: there would be no more moments, there had never been any. It was eternity, an eternity of fear and distress. The ultimate reality that the mystics talk about, and that Hervé and I talked about while hiking in the Valais region, was this: this painting by Raoul Dufy and the infinite badness ema-nating from these women in hoop dresses and children in sailor suits. I'd seen what should not be seen: the bottom of the barrel. And, as in some nightmares I had as a child, which sent me hurtling to damnation, like the snakes in Snakes and Ladders, I heard a voice say calmly and kindly in my ear—this kindness was the worst thing of all: "You've arrived. You're here. You didn't know it, but in fact you've always been here. You told yourself this long, complicated story that you call your life, a story about how you were born, had parents, went to school, knew people, traveled, learned foreign languages, read and wrote books, loved women, caressed their bodies—which is what you loved the most—had children, did yoga, shat and pissed, were happy sometimes, suffered more because that's what you're like, made others suffer because that's also what you're like, and then a moment comes when this long story full of characters and events that you call your life winds up here. The place of endless distress, of the bottomless pit, of the weeping and gnashing of teeth, where your neighbor in the secure unit screams. The end of the line. You're back. We've been waiting for you.

"You're here."

ECT

"Significant thymic decline with intolerable moral suffering, feelings of distress and incurability, numerous bouts of tears, impression of bradypsychia." You pick up vocabulary in a psychiatric ward: bradypsychia is the slowing down of thought, and in addition to my intolerable moral suffering I must have been slowed down quite a lot for the medical team to decide to use the heavy artillery, that is, what used to be called electroshocks and is now called ECT, or electroconvulsive therapy. This change of name is intended to make people forget the archaic and barbaric reputation of a treatment that immediately brings to mind scenes from *One Flew Over the Cuckoo's Nest*. After having been practically abandoned—also due to this reputation—it's been more in use once again since the nineties. These artificial epileptic seizures are meant to cause a sort of "reset" in patients, and are today considered a leading-edge treatment, recommended for severe depression and certain types of schizophrenia. Nevertheless, resorting to them is still a difficult decision, and one the patient is generally unable to make by himself: that was my case. If psychiatrists then leave the decision to the patients' relatives, it's because they firmly believe that this is the way to go. They even go so far as saying that it's all they have to offer. We've reached the end, if we want to save him it's this or nothing. François Samuelson, who's been my agent and friend for the past thirty years, was Nathalie's main contact at the time, and he told me about the hours of anguish they went through before finally saying: okay, if we haven't got a choice, you know what you're doing, go ahead. But really, was there no other choice? Would I have made it through without ECT? How would I have fared? What would my life have been like if instead of going to the Sainte-Anne Psychiatric Hospital and waking up fourteen times in a row in front of the atrocious poster for the Dufy exhibition, I had left—in pieces, fine, but nevertheless left—for Iraq? I don't know, and I'll never know. You can never know what would have happened if you'd taken another direction. Sometimes I think that the danger and adrenaline would have given me back a taste for life, other times that the alternative wasn't "ECT or Iraq" but "ECT or death." That's also what the psychiatrist who's continued to treat me since then, and in whom I have great confidence, thinks. He's seen a lot of melancholic depressives in his time. He knows how to assess the risk of suicide, which he considered to be very high in my case, and I myself realize on rereading these pages that I can find no words to adequately convey the "intolerable moral suffering" mentioned in my medical report. If I can find no words, it's because I'm too distant and detached today to be able to remember, describe, or name the horror in which I was then immersed, and above all, I think, because there are no words for it. What I'm saying here sounds horrible, but in fact it was much more horrible than that. It was an unspeakable, indescribable, unqualifiable, and—the word hardly exists, but no matter— immemorable horror. When you're no longer there, you can no longer remember *that*—thank goodness. So yes, maybe the ECT did save my life. But whatever the case, the improvement wasn't spectacular. All during the treatment, my hospital report speaks of "nonlinear development with moments of thymic improvement, without a clear recovery of vitality," "significant thymic decline with anxiety and negative thoughts," and "increasing memory problems." Ah yes, the increasing memory problems . . . We'll have to talk about that, let's do it.

"Increasing memory problems"

In my experience, these memory lapses are the major— and most serious—side effect of ECT. You're told that they're temporary, that your memory will come back, that at most the loss will last only as long as the treatment period, but it's not true. I'm writing these pages three years after the fact, and my memory is still a field of ruins. A few days ago I chanced to hear a cover of Jacques Brel's "La

Chanson des vieux amants" by the American singer Melody Gardot, which I liked so much that I tried to find out more about Melody Gardot. The first thing I read was an interview where she says that in the wake of a terrible accident she suffers from short-term and long-term memory loss to such an extent that starting each day is like climbing Mount Everest. Before she gets up, she has to collect as many memories as she can, not only about what she's got to do in the next few hours and what she did the previous day, but about her entire past, and even her identity. For her it's an effort to remember her name, her age, and the main events in her life. Okay, I'm not there yet, nevertheless it often happens to me that I talk to a friend without remembering what we said the day before, or even that we spoke the day before. I'm constantly afraid that the people I love will think I'm either neglectful or inattentive, or that I have the beginnings of Alzheimer's—which wouldn't be unlikely, because like the risk of suicide, the risk of Alzheimer's is twenty times higher than average among people with bipolar disorder. There is, however, a silver lining to all of this, because if memory loss is the collateral damage of electroshocks, they also had a totally unexpected collateral benefit, which is that I started memorizing poetry.

I learn poetry

One day, in the cafeteria of Sainte-Anne, where he'd come to join me for a hot chocolate, I complained about these memory problems to my friend Olivier Rubenstein. He said:

"You should memorize poetry, that'll take the rust off your neurons." Personally, I've never been a reader of poetry. In fact, even though I've regretted it, all my life I've believed I was completely closed to verse. But then Olivier brought me Jean-François Revel's marvelous anthology of French poetry, which I'd owned for decades practically without ever having opened it, ever since the days when we used to see its author pushing his cart full of wine bottles at the supermarket in Paimpol. And in this horribly difficult time, it made my life more bearable. What makes it marvelous is that it's neither an honor list nor the result of a consensus, but an expression of the particular, absolutely independent taste of a man who, listening only to his inner voice, could include just one verse by a hugely famous poet while retaining *everything* that the sixteenth-century poet Louise Labé left to posterity—a handful of sonnets testifying to incandescent, unrequited passion. I subsequently learned many other poems, but the very first was precisely this sonnet by her—a choice that, after everything I've just told, I don't think I need to justify:

> I live, I die, I burn, I drown
> I endure at once chill and cold
> Life is at once too soft and too hard
> I have sore troubles mingled with joys.
>
> Suddenly I laugh and at the same time cry
> And in pleasure many a grief endure
> My happiness wanes and yet it lasts unchanged
> All at once I dry up and grow green.

Thus I suffer love's inconstancies
And when I think the pain is most intense
Without thinking, it is gone again.

Then when I feel my joys certain
And my hour of greatest delight arrived
I find my pain beginning all over once again.

"Good transient recovery . . ."

I'm discharged from Sainte-Anne at the end of April, and the report ends with this observation: "Good transient recovery but frequent relapses." The fact is that for at least three months I've been doing better, much better even. The medication seems to be working. The psychiatrists authorize my departure for Iraq, where my report with Lucas will very much resemble what it's been until now, that is, the drowsy hours we spent at the Iraqi consulate on Avenue Foch all last winter. Just like in Paris, in Baghdad we'll sit on deep, hideous sofas and sip small glasses of very strong, very sweet, very delicious tea, until after several hours of waiting we'll be ushered into the office of a high dignitary, ulama or ayatollah, Shiite or Sunni, who'll spool off endless politico-religious cant. From one high dignitary to the next, we'll drive in an armored jeep between the concrete walls that surround and protect all the buildings in Baghdad from car bombs and make it a completely walled city. There's no tangible threat, no obvious danger: in that respect I'm a little disappointed. We won't find the

Blood Quran. Its trace is lost in the famous mosque with the Kalashnikov-shaped minarets where it was displayed until it was transferred to some unknown location, probably in Saudi Arabia. As the subject of our investigation shifts gradually from Saddam to his mysterious calligrapher, who also seems to have taken refuge in Saudi Arabia, Lucas and I resolve to follow up our report in that country, and above all to rekindle the complicity that made our stay in a city as unpleasant as Baghdad so pleasant—Iraq being, after all, the archetype of what Donald Trump, in his charming language, called "a shithole country."

". . . but rapid relapses"

Summer arrives, we take up residence on the beautiful island of Patmos, where we have a house at the foot of the Monastery of Saint John the Theologian, who's supposed to have written the book of Revelation there. In my ideal picture of what a serene life and radiant maturity would look like, Patmos plays the role of Homer's Ithaca. But this time as soon as I set foot on the island from which I expected a peaceful, soothing routine, something happens to me that eludes and frightens me. I try to hide it, above all from myself. Everyone has passing clouds, nothing to worry about. However, I do worry about something, and this worry feeds on itself. I'm afraid the madness will return. I'm afraid I'll be the plaything of some inner monster, over whom I have no control. I'm afraid that a sudden, unhabitual burst of aggression will announce a manic crisis.

I'm afraid of the depression that will come in its wake. I'm afraid of the subterranean effects of the drugs I've been prescribed, which may be changing me without my knowing. The harmony of Patmos to which I'd been so looking forward begins to weigh on me. It starts getting on my nerves. I like vacations only if I can work, at least a little. After a bit of yoga on the terrace, I like to leave the house at sunrise and go write in the only café already open in the village. I'm the only customer. When others start to arrive, I leave and go to the bakery to buy pastries, which I bring home for a breakfast that stretches, what with people getting up at different times and successive pots of tea and coffee, late into the morning. I loved these joyful, relaxed rituals, I loved it when our friends came to join us under the pergola, I loved playing the generous host. But now I feel like a stranger in our own home, a keyed-up, irritable stranger. Although I take my folder of notes on yoga with me every morning, I've got nothing to write in the café, nothing to say to the café owner, to whom I normally enjoy talking, nothing to say to our friends. I no longer feel like reciting all the verses by Ronsard or La Fontaine, Apollinaire or Yves Bonnefoy that I've doggedly been trying to learn in the hopes of curbing my anxiety, and that don't curb anything at all. Here is Ronsard:

> *We must leave behind houses and orchards and gardens,*
> *Dishes and vessels which the artisan engraved,*
> *On to the final rites, much like the swan*
> *Whose death song is sung by Meander's water.*

> *It is done: I have unwound the threads of my fate.*
> *I have lived, I have made my name rather remarkable . . .*

Today I couldn't care less about making my name rather remarkable. Everything that's ever mattered to me, everything I've dreamed of, glory and mansions, love and wisdom, has lost all meaning. I'm going around in circles, one moment I'm listless, the next I can't stand still. And it's the start of what people are calling the refugee crisis. You can't say that we hear much about it on Patmos, but hundreds, thousands of migrants from Afghanistan, Eritrea, Somalia, and above all Bashar al-Assad's smoldering Syria flock to the Greek coast every day. The peaceful Dodecanese Islands, just a stone's throw from Turkey, selectively take them in. The more upscale ones like ours are spared by what the inhabitants and summer sojourners agree—without saying it too loudly—is a plague, while the less trendy islands like Leros and Lesbos take in more than their share. Our friend Laurence de Cambronne, who used to work as a journalist before she came to live on Patmos for six months out of every year, has gone to Leros on assignment. She comes over to our place for dinner, talks about the situation, gets worked up and then indignant. She evokes the courage of the migrants, the indifference of some of the inhabitants, the dedication of others, and an American historian who's left everything to do a wonderful job over there. Listening to her, we're a little ashamed of our carefree life, the life of the blessed of the world, dressed in elegantly crinkled white linen and having little more to do than decide what beach to hit, based on which tavern it's near and how the wind is blowing. I think to myself that Baghdad did me a world of good, and that on this nearby island where serious things are happening, fate may be offering me a second chance to get away from myself. So the next morning I go down to the harbor with a bag containing some clothes and my notes on yoga and, unaware that I'm leaving our Ithaca forever, I board the ferry to Leros, where Frederica Mojave awaits me.

IV

THE BOYS

Frederica

It was impossible to miss her on the quay. She's very tall—at least six feet—and powerfully built, with an angular, ungraceful face that I immediately find noble. In her sixties, with a thick mane of gray hair, she's wearing a midnight-blue dress that's far too dressy for a Greek island in midsummer, and she greets me brusquely, without suggesting that we have coffee or even asking after Laurence, who put the two of us in touch. Her creative writing workshop starts in half an hour, there's no time to lose. She almost runs to the scooter rental place, with me tagging along behind her. The first thing you do on a Greek island is rent a scooter; the deal is quickly closed, but I'm surprised when Frederica climbs on behind me. She lives on Leros all year round and doesn't have a scooter? Or a car? How does she manage? "I manage," she replies, annoyed, and off we drive, with her guiding me. At first sight, Leros is very different from

Patmos and the other Greek islands I know. The houses aren't photogenic assemblages of white cubes with blue shutters, but modernist villas. Remnants, I'd later learn, of the Italian occupation in the 1930s. They're now dilapidated, with cracked walls and abandoned gardens. We also pass large neoclassical buildings lining piazzas drawn with a compass: too big, too circular, too empty. Under the leaden sun, they're reminiscent of Giorgio de Chirico's metaphysical paintings. Huge roots break through the road, on which mangy-looking dogs lie sleeping. Frederica must have sensed my astonishment. From behind me she leans over my shoulder: "It's Africa here." Africa maybe, but it reminds me more of San Clemente, the island near Venice that for more than a century was a vast insane asylum, and about which Raymond Depardon and Sophie Ristelhueber shot a gripping documentary. Speaking of which, we pass the psychiatric hospital, a vast complex of pavilions built to accommodate the insane from all over the Dodecanese. Most of the buildings have now been transformed into a hot spot, that is, a refugee camp. From the dusty road we see containers, barbed wire, police. There isn't a single tree on this part of the island, not the slightest shade. "There are a thousand people in there," Frederica shouts in my ear, "but we're not allowed in." When you arrive from elegant, peaceful Patmos, these almost warlike images are surprising. I don't have a very clear idea about what's going on here: my own personal meltdown has left me little time to follow the refugee crisis, and I have only a vague understanding of the agreement signed a few months earlier between Turkey and the European Union. If I came here, it's because I'm looking for a place I can go when I no longer know where I can go, and I feel like I've found it.

At the Pikpa

The so-called Pikpa is an imposing edifice, also strongly influenced by Mussolinian architecture. Like many buildings on the island, it was an annex of the psychiatric hospital and has now been converted hurriedly into a reception center for migrants. When you enter the large hall you think that although it's not paradise, those who arrive are nonetheless lucky to end up here and not in the containers of the fenced-off hot spot under the blazing sun. It's clean, bright, well aired. Children laugh and play and chase one another around. Young people from all over Europe look after them. A schedule posted in the hall announces language classes (Greek, English, German), as well as courses on gardening, cooking, yoga, and creative writing, the one taught by Frederica. It takes place in a classroom that doubles as a dormitory. There are bunk beds and makeshift curtains that give as much privacy as possible and, in the middle, two tables where our students sit waiting patiently: four teenagers dressed in very clean T-shirts and jeans—none of them wear shorts, unlike three quarters of the people here. The room is also very clean, there's nothing on the floor—perhaps because they're tidy, but mostly because they don't have much stuff. Frederica introduces me as Emmanuel, a French writer who's come to share his competence—that's what she says in English: "to share his competence." As she says it she turns her head sharply to the left, as if someone had called her, as if she was looking for someone or something on her left, but no one's called her, there's no one on her left. When she turns to us again, her face remains worried for a few moments. Her students seem used to this tic, which happens to her often, maybe every five minutes or so. I'll soon get used to it too. After that, she asks everyone to introduce themselves in turn. Going clockwise around the room, there's Hamid, a handsome, serious-looking boy, Afghan, seventeen; Atiq, less handsome but with an open, smiling face, also Afghan, also seventeen; Mohamed, who's Pakistani, not as good-looking and more timid, sixteen; and finally Hassan, Afghan, the youngest at fifteen. Frederica concludes the round by introducing herself, for my benefit only as she's been working with the four teenagers for several weeks already. "I'm Frederica," she says, "but people call me either Fred or Erica, so you can take your pick." I say, "Okay, I'll call you Erica." The boys laugh, Erica does too. I ask why, and Atiq explains that while Hamid and he have chosen to call Frederica Fred, Mohamed and Hassan call her Erica, and this small conflict amuses them a lot: it's as if instead of one teacher they had two, with different characters. Atiq talks to me directly. He looks straight at me, tries to get my attention, he's the only one who speaks good English. Erica adds that she's American, that she's from Boise, Idaho, where she was a medieval history teacher, and that she now lives on Leros, where she also shares her competence. She only speaks English, not Greek, never mind the Farsi spoken by Hamid, Atiq, and Hassan or the Urdu spoken by

Mohamed. In the two months they've been here together, Atiq has been teaching the other three English. Only Hamid has really benefited from these lessons, so the two of them act as interpreters for Mohamed and Hassan. The four met in the big Moria refugee camp on Lesbos, Hamid tells me, and they thank their lucky stars that they were sent to Leros together. Together they form a gang, almost a family, and nothing is more precious on a journey like theirs. They can rely on one another, they're afraid of being separated. At the same time, Atiq adds, still talking directly to me, they know very well that they will be separated, and it would be nice if at least two of them could stay together. It's both moving and cruel to see how Atiq, at just seventeen, refuses to delude himself, how he knows that life is a machine for separating people. What's also moving and cruel, which I guessed and Erica confirms, is that Atiq and Hamid like Mohamed and Hassan, but if it comes down to only two of them being able to stay together, if only two of them are clever enough not to let life separate them, it'll be Atiq and Hamid. Too bad for the other two, who are less well equipped for survival. During the class, which lasts an hour and a half without anyone showing signs of fatigue, I observe them both. Hamid is remarkably handsome, with fine features and velvety, melancholy black eyes. Atiq is rather unattractive, his face ravaged by acne and the beginnings of a double chin, but he's got charisma and vitality on his side, he's the natural leader, he's the one who'll start bringing girls back to their place—or who's already bringing girls back to their place—no, that would surprise me, the four of them are certainly virgins.

"The night before I left"

Frederica asked the boys to work on the topic "The night before I left." Not surprisingly, Atiq is the first to hand in his assignment. He's written and printed up two pages of text in the Pikpa offices. He reads them aloud, warning us that he won't start with the last night but with the night before that. It was in Quetta, Pakistan, where he'd gone to live with his aunt and her husband after his parents died when he was very young. That evening he'd smoked a hookah with some friends. They'd had a good time, joked around, he was feeling good. Atiq is sociable, it's important for him to have good friends, guys he can count on and who can count on him. He came home quite late, his aunt and her husband should have been in bed a long time ago, but they were waiting for him at the entrance to the building. He thought they were worried and angry because he'd come home so late, and that they were going to tell him off. No: they were waiting to tell him that he was going to leave for Europe in two days. The agreement was made with his uncle who works as a cook in Belgium, and who organized and paid for the trip. Atiq had been told nothing about this arrangement. Everything was done for his own good, but behind his back, and he feels cheated. He says so. His adoptive parents are troubled, as if they hadn't expected this reaction. The next morning, the last morning of his normal life, his aunt gives him fifty dollars to buy clothes for the trip: jeans, T-shirts. She seems to think this will sweeten the pill. Buying these clothes is all the easier because his uncle manages the department store downstairs.

Atiq goes down, walks around the shop, but he's so sad that he doesn't buy or even try on a thing. For a moment he thinks he'll go visit his friends and say goodbye to them one by one, maybe use the fifty dollars to invite them all for a last get-together like the one they had the night before. But they'd have a terrible time, he realizes. If he thought he'd see them again it'd be easy, they could enjoy themselves. But now they'd all know they'll probably never see one another again, so what could they say? It'd be too sad, it's too sad. All he does is visit his parents' graves to say goodbye. Then he describes the dinner with his aunt and his family. The food tastes funny, he can't eat. It's very strange because it seems like a normal evening, they talk about normal things, not about his departure, and yet he's going to leave at four o'clock in the morning, at sixteen years old, forever. His aunt comes to his room to help him pack his bag. It's a sports bag, he usually puts his tennis stuff in it, the handle of his racket sticks out. He plays well, and wonders if he should take the racket with him. When he goes to do it, his aunt takes it out of the bag and puts it in the cupboard, without a word. She's surprised, annoyed even, that he didn't spend the fifty dollars she'd given him on clothes. Otherwise he's got what he needs, two hundred dollars in a money belt. He should take his fleece jacket, his aunt says, it'll be cold on the way. When she folds the fleece and tucks it in the bag, Atiq suddenly starts crying like a child. Rather than hug him, she talks to him seriously, as if he were an adult. He remembers her exact words: "Stop crying, my boy. In life you have to leave everything, always, and in the end it's life you have to leave, so

there's no use crying, don't cry." Atiq spends the last hours
wandering around his childhood home, pushing open the
doors of rooms that no longer look the way they used to.
He feels—I noted the flurry of adjectives—confused/sad/
angry/lonely. It's no longer his house, but already the house
as it will be the next day, the house he'll have left, the
house without him. After this Atiq falls silent, indicating
that the story is over. Erica twists her neck as far as she
can to the left. When she comes back to us she murmurs:
"It's so hard . . . There's so much grief . . . So much . . ."
The way she says it rings true, her emotion rings true, and
I feel a huge amount of sympathy for her. Atiq then points
to Hassan, whom until now I've only heard say his name,
and says: "It was hard, but it was even harder for Hassan.
Because he had no one to say goodbye to. No one helped
him pack his bag." Silence. Hassan looks uneasily at Atiq.
He understands that Atiq was just talking about him,
but doesn't know what he said. Finally Hamid leans over
and translates. Hassan then takes his head in his hands
and starts banging it on the table, moaning loudly. We all
freeze, but Erica, who's next to him, puts her arm around
his shoulders, hugs him, rocks him in her arms, and calms
his tears: "Hassan, Hassan, I'm here, we're here, we're together. We're like a little family, you've all been so brave,
you're all so brave . . ." Then we all start putting our hands
on Hassan to comfort him, some on his shoulder, some on
his arm. I run my hand through his hair. It's an unusually
intimate gesture, but it comes naturally and seems to me
quite normal when I do it.

Michael Haneke

Lunch is served in the playground, chicken with rice
served in aluminum trays. Everything's quite cheerful.
Children play soccer or hopscotch—it seems like ages
since I've seen children play hopscotch. The volunteers
look like summer camp counselors. There are two pretty
Italian twin sisters. An anorexic Irishwoman with tattoos
all over her body teaches children how to make costume
jewelry with paper clips and wire hangers, and a little Eri-
trean girl shows me hers with a smile that could be used
to define the word *radiant*. Everyone is young, with the exception of an Austrian couple. The man is blind in one eye
and also has a pleasant, somewhat evangelical smile, while
his wife is thickset, jaunty, and loud. Until their retirement
they worked as archaeologists, and, they say with a laugh,
giving me the feeling it's an often-repeated joke, they speak
modern Greek poorly but ancient Greek well, and it's surprising how far that'll get you. They did most of their fieldwork in Syria, and if they now devote part of their vacation
to volunteering, it's to return some of the magnificent hos-
pitality the Syrians have shown them. She, Elfriede, blares
at me how impressed she is with the Greeks' dedication
and how ashamed she is of her country for not even honor-
ing its commitment to take in 37,500 refugees, a figure she
considers obscenely low. Listening with waning interest to
her tirade on the immigration policies of the host countries
and the conflicting goals of the European Union, I watch
out of the corner of my eye as her husband, the evangelical

Moritz, sits at a small kindergarten table under a tree with a six- or seven-year-old boy he's helping with his drawing. The boy, who I later learn is Syrian and named Elias, refuses to put the cap back on the felt pen he's been using, and drops it on the ground. Moritz says that he's got all the time in the world, and that if the boy wants to drop the cap, fine, he'll make him to pick it up a hundred times, a thousand, if necessary. He says this in a calm but increasingly curt and menacing tone, and it's difficult to know whether this is a game the child is enjoying or a display of sadistic firmness right out of a Michael Haneke film.

My profile photo

It's easy to find a place to stay on the Greek islands. I haven't booked anything, and when I ask Erica if there's somewhere she can recommend, she replies with her usual brusqueness that I should just come and stay with her: she's got a big house with a guest room, that'll make working together easier. Located above the port where I landed and quite far from the sea, Erica's house is neither a white-and-blue cube nor a specimen of fascist architecture, but a building from the seventies in keeping with the taste of the Greek middle class at the time, that is to say ugly. Only her bedroom upstairs has a view of the harbor and a small stretch of blue sea. The living room on the ground floor is windowless and all but empty, and the guest room where I'll stay is a child's bedroom/storeroom with a tiny bed that's barely big enough for one person and piles of boxes that still haven't been unpacked. In five minutes I could have found a room in the port that was ten times nicer, but it's too late to change my mind. Erica has already handed me a pair of unmatching sheets and a scratchy towel, and offers me coffee, which we drink on the terrace behind the house, it too without a view. She also says I can take a shower, which I refuse, even though in this heat no one misses the opportunity to take one, especially after a trip and a busy day, but these days I get a macabre pleasure from steeping in my nervous sweat and stinky clothes. I've also started smoking again, and when I smoke it's like when I drink: I do it a lot. We're still reeling from the class, from Atiq's story and especially from the violence with which he laid bare Hassan's distress. Hassan has nothing. He's completely alone. He's the youngest of the group, the only one without a smartphone. And in their situation that's the worst thing that can happen. The others at least have this way of communicating, everything they own is in the memory of their smartphone, losing it is a catastrophe. They're very active on Facebook, and Erica reads their posts every day. She shows me some on her phone. Atiq: "You know the difference between *like* and *love*? If you *like* a flower, you pick it. If you *love* it, you water it. Whoever has understood that has understood life." I wonder if this is a well-known jingle, like: "'Give a man a fish and he will eat for a day. Teach a man to fish and you feed him for a lifetime,'" or if Atiq came up with it on his own. I've never heard it before, neither has Erica. A post from Hamid, now, under a selfie where he's impressively handsome, as handsome as the young Alain Delon, I'm not kidding: "Behind my smile my heart is bleeding. The face you see is that of

a lost boy." Three weeks earlier Hamid had posted pictures
of himself in a hospital bed and his slashed wrist, after he
tried to commit suicide with a razor. Atiq, too, who seems
so positive, so dynamic, has terrible bouts of despondency.
They all have them, they all feel so alone in the world that
at one point or another they think it's no longer worth putting up a fight, that it's better to die. Erica asks if I have a
Facebook account. Yes, I've just opened one, Laurence told
me that it was indispensable if I was going to have deal-
ings with refugees. My daughter Jeanne, who was ten at
the time, helped me with it, and even though she wasn't in
such a good mood that day, she burst out laughing when I
had to upload a "profile photo" and showed her my profile
so she could take a picture. I tell Erica the story and, now
that I'm being witty, I follow it up with another about my
yoga teacher, Toni, who barked "Hold your calves" during
a class, and one student actually bent down and grabbed
his calves with his hands. The rest of us all cracked up, because the idea wasn't to do it literally, of course, but to hold
your calves *from the inside*, mentally. The story seemed
very funny to me when I started telling it, but by the time I
get to the end some thirty seconds later I feel not only like
it's a complete flop, but also that I'm displaying my mental
collapse as unrelentingly as Atiq revealed Hassan's almost
metaphysical misfortune. But instead of looking at me in
dismay, Erica laughs heartily too. The stress that seems to
dog her vanishes, and she asks me what kind of yoga I do.
Iyengar? She does Ashtanga, and if I want to practice she
has a mat that she can lend me. One yoga mat for two, one
scooter for two: Erica and I are already becoming a couple.

Toxic meditation

Is meditation possible when you're fraught with anxiety, you smoke two packs of cigarettes a day, and your mind is a steady flow of toxic thoughts: regret, remorse, resentment, and fear of abandonment? When there's nowhere you can take refuge and you're entirely at the mercy of the very worst in you? Possible or not, I try it at siesta time in Erica's children's room. The shutters are closed, but I can hear quiet noises outside: a broom swept unhurriedly, water running in a house nearby, a cat meowing, a scooter backfiring in the distance, the hum of a refrigerator. I try to focus my attention on them, and on the faint sound of breath in my nostrils: irregular, wheezy, choked. I try not to move, to remain completely still. Not moving is hard work. Even if you're unaware of it, even when it's imperceptible, you're actually moving all the time—hardly less so than those annoying people who cross their legs then don't stop wiggling their foot in the air. Not moving at all requires a huge amount of concentration. To make it easier I use a yoga technique: pushing the outside of myself inward, and the inside outward. The skin toward the muscles, the muscles toward the bones, the bones toward the marrow. And inversely: the marrow toward the surface of the bones, the bones toward the muscles, the muscles toward the skin. Expansion and contraction, centrifugal and centripetal movement, at the same time. The butter and the money for the butter. Even if it takes a bit of imagination when it comes to the marrow, I manage to hold myself in this vise and, thus entrapped, stop myself from getting up to smoke another cigarette, which is both the symptom of and the fuel for my anxiety. Even though I'm sitting stock-still like this, you can't say that I want to smoke any less, that the toxic thoughts are calmed, or that my anxiety is less intense. You can't say I see things more clearly. You can't say I can put my suffering in perspective. No, you can't say any of that, and when I think back on all the fine definitions of meditation I thought I'd list over the course of my upbeat, subtle little book on yoga, they don't make me upbeat, let alone subtly upbeat, but rather snide and bitter. Nonetheless, sitting in the lotus position for half an hour as I've just done in Erica's guest room, I feel, if not relief, at least a sense of being sheltered. That doesn't stop the dreadful flux of thoughts, but at least it can stop me from fidgeting. It's not much, but it does a bit of good. I know that when I straighten out my legs it'll be to go get a cigarette, anxiously check my tablet, and write an email that, although it tries to clear things up, will only make them worse. So I put off the moment before this programmed debacle. I wait a bit more. I stay a little longer out of harm's way.

Nothing in the cupboards

At the end of the afternoon, Erica knocks on my door and asks if I want to have a drink on the terrace. I do, so I have to go with her to the corner shop to get what we need. I understand that from now on we'll do everything together. Our shopping list is basic: a bottle of white wine, some olives, a bag of pistachios. This house with nothing in it—not a bottle in the fridge or a box of crackers in the cupboard—is a picture of rare desolation: the very opposite of a well-kept house where a family lives, where the fridge is full, where you're always ready to welcome friends over a big impromptu dish of pasta. I've been living in such a house for years, I'm busy extracting myself from it, and I'm terrified that I'll soon be living in what's at best a better-off version of this one, in which Erica feels good, as she valiantly maintains, but which oozes the cruelest loneliness, and which even in midsummer you can sense will be stone-cold come September. Although my capacity for interest in others is at a real low at the moment, Erica intrigues me. How did she end up here? What's her story? I ask her straight out, uncorking the bottle of white wine. She waits for me to fill our glasses, raises hers, and answers just as directly: "Failure in love, the story of my life." In a nutshell: she'd just retired from her chair in medieval history at Boise State University in Idaho when she met a Dutch jazz bassist on a trip to Amsterdam and fell in love with him—a love so mutual, it seemed, that he swept her away to Leros, where after a few weeks they bought this house together. They planned to live there half the year and in Amsterdam the other half, it could have been a wonderful life, but they didn't live together in either Leros or Amsterdam because without warning the Dutch bass player ran off with another woman and is now demanding either that they sell the house or that Erica buy his share, which she can't afford. This last point surprises me a little, because in my view half of such an unattractive house, far from the sea, on an island that's not very popular with tourists, can't be out of reach for a retired American academic. Whatever the financial reasons for her plight, Erica finds herself trapped on this island where she knows no one and can only get around by taxi, since she can't drive a scooter and is afraid to learn. That, she sums up with robust humor, is how to become the ideal volunteer and drown your sorrows in altruism.

"A subtle flavor of asshole"

The bottle emptied, we go for dinner at a tavern in the port. The wind has picked up, the blusterous *meltem*, which is the Greek version of the French mistral. It blows sand on our grilled fish, knocks over tables, and gusts so hard that we can hardly hear each other, but tonight Erica wants to talk. I listen as best I can to what she shouts over to me about how the retsina we're drinking is made, about the disgusting chemicals with which all wines, even the best, are cut nowadays, and about how the dictatorship of the U.S. wine critic Robert Parker has done such a disservice to the great Bordeaux . . . This almost fundamentalist rant clashes with what I observe in her way of drinking, which is very close to mine: quality, schmality—any plonk will do, what counts is getting drunk. Russian style. I make her laugh, with a laugh that must be pleasantly wicked for her, by vehemently explaining that wine criticism disgusts me and that I hate people who, as they say, *savor* wine, swirling it for ages in huge glasses before discerning woody notes or a subtle flavor of asshole. I actually said that, "a subtle flavor of asshole," in my despair I was quite cheerful that night. After ordering another bottle of wine, the third that evening, Erica asks a question that surprises and amuses me: If we were speaking French, would we be saying *tu* or *vous* to each other? I answer that at this very moment, right here at this table, we'd probably be deciding to switch from *vous* to *tu*. The bottle arrives, I fill our glasses, we drink to our calling each other *tu* and our newfound friendship. It's too bad that distinction doesn't exist in English, Erica says, because people's preference for the informal *tu* or the more formal *vous* says a lot about them. It's the same, she adds, without the connection being very clear to me, for people who swim parallel to the beach and those who swim perpendicular to it, out to sea. "I swim out to sea," she says. After a moment's thought, I say that I do too, and she nods in satisfaction: she's not surprised. I feel like I've passed a test: if I'd swum parallel to the shore that would have been it between Erica and me. And then, she continues, there are the people who turn off the light when they leave a room and those who don't, the people who take the elevator downstairs and those who don't even understand that you can do such a thing, the people who give money to beggars and those who don't, the people who cede to temptation and read the diary of the person they love if they come across it and those who don't, the people who act the same way whether someone is watching or not and those who act differently when they're being watched. This last distinction strikes me, the way you can be struck by something that's obvious but that had never struck you as obvious until now. I haven't read Kant, but from the little

I know of him that could be a Kantian thing: acting the same way whether someone's watching or not seems to me like the cornerstone of morality. We agree on this point, we're happy to agree, we definitely agree on a lot of things, and throughout dinner, almost yelling, we get a kick out of drawing up a list of the divided classes of humanity: those who see the glass as half empty and those who see it as half full, those who vote Democrat and those who vote Republican, those who prefer Dostoyevsky and those who prefer Tolstoy—in the French version it's Voltaire and Rousseau, in the American Faulkner and Hemingway— those who, when they're in someone else's kitchen, figure out for themselves where things go and put them away without asking, and those who stand around and ask, "Is there something I can do?" There, I admit that I belong to the second category. On that note, I ask her what she knows about yin and yang, the poles that are at the heart of Chinese thought. Not much, a little more than the journalist who interviewed me about yoga, and once I've cited a few obvious examples like the perennial day/night, hot/ cold, attack/defense, active/passive, inhale/exhale, even/odd, we start looking for more unexpected ones. She caught on fast: once it had been established that concave is yin and convex is yang, she said that cock is yang and pussy is yin— those are my words: I think I remember her saying *penis* and *vagina*, two words I personally find it difficult to use. Pee is yin, we go on, and poo is yang; reading is yin, writing is yang; poetry is yin, prose is yang; what unfolds in time is yin, what unfolds in space is yang; so music is yin and painting is yang. What's below is yin, what's above is yang;

the back is yin, the front is yang; half is yin, the whole
is yang—I'm the one who says that, so I can place Hesiod's saying, which of course I got from Hervé: "The half
is greater than the whole." Erica is amazed by Hesiod's
brilliant phrase and repeats it with respect: "The half is
greater than the whole . . ." Then it's my turn to be amazed
when she replies that losing is yin and winning is yang, but
that losing is the best way to win. "It suits the two of us
to think that way, right?" Every four or five minutes, Erica
cranes her neck as far as she can to the left to search for
her words, and it's from one of these expeditions behind
herself that she brings back this ultimate distinction between two species of humanity: those who call her Fred
and those who call her Erica. Why did I choose Erica over
Fred? I realize that it says a lot about me, but I have to admit that I don't have an answer.

The "Heroic" Polonaise

When we get home, not without buying a fourth bottle at
the tavern, it's too windy to sit out on the terrace so we
retreat to the windowless living room. As I open our last
bottle, wondering if it wouldn't have been wiser to buy two
instead, Erica rummages through her collection of CDs
and slips one into her big old boom box. Piano music. A
peal of arpeggios. I don't play an instrument or read notes,
unfortunately, but I love music and know it well enough.
When I listen to the classical radio station France Musique,
mostly in the car, I take childish pride in identifying most

of the works in the first few bars. Erica shoots me a defiant look, impatient and imperious, as if she knew I had this social talent and was giving me a challenge, which I take up with panache. Chopin: Chopin's most famous polonaise, the "Heroic" Polonaise. Bang on. Erica is over the moon. To be honest, this great epic edifice isn't my favorite work by Chopin, far from it, nevertheless tonight I'm transported by its grandeur, its majesty, and I thank Erica effusively for putting on precisely this piece at precisely this time: nothing could be more appropriate. I ask who's playing. Vladimir Horowitz, she says as proudly as if it were her, and it's an interpretation of mad, diabolical virtuosity. When you hear it, you dream of being in his shoes and unleashing with your own fingers these sonic cataclysms, punctuated by moments of plaintive reverie. We listen to the piece, standing together in the middle of the living room. Erica knows it by heart, and signals to me when the passages she loves the most are coming up, the ones that give her goose bumps and lift her to the skies, and I wonder how, loving Chopin as I do, I've managed to neglect the "Heroic" Polonaise until I was almost sixty, with its incredible rhythmic power, sumptuous octave crescendos, and ever more grandiose returns of the main theme—the first interlude like a fantastic horse ride, and the second like a gracefully uncoiled garland, pure Chopin, weightless and magical. When the piece is finished, Erica puts it back on without asking, but there's no need to ask, and the second time I appreciate all the more the bits that hit me the first time like a Steinway falling from the tenth floor. Enthused by my enthusiasm, Erica takes my arm and says: "Listen,

listen, that little note!" And yes, once you've heard it, all you want to do is hear it again, that little note suspended in the air, that little D natural—I can tell you now but I didn't know it then—all alone, fragile, a distant star from which the garland will miraculously unfurl. We listen to the garland unfold. Clearly, Chopin loves it so much that he doesn't want to let it go so he starts again, resuming the melody a little higher, embellishing it with trills, we want it to last forever but we know that the main theme, the great heroic theme, will come back and that it will be even more beautiful, even more climactic if that's possible, and when it does, *maestoso*, topping off our joy, I start waving my arms and, although for me at this moment I'm a blend of Horowitz and von Karajan, my gesticulations must be more like those of Boris Yeltsin when, totally drunk at a ceremony where he was Helmut Kohl's guest of honor, he lurched to his feet and staggered toward the military band, took the conductor's baton from his hand, and started wiggling it, filling the vast majority of his compatriots with shame despite their willingness to indulge all things alcohol-related. Erica and I are now dancing in the living room, if you can call the mixture of bear waddling and tai chi movements that I do—which literally have her wailing with laughter—dancing. When the music takes her and she moves to it—as badly and elatedly as I do—Erica's tic disappears. Effusive as always after I drink, I repeat to her in a slurred voice that we're now friends because in the depths of our despair we've listened to Polonaise No. 6, the "Heroic," together, so we're necessarily friends, great friends. As soon as it's over Erica puts it right back to the beginning. There

are other magnificent works in this two-CD set by Vladimir Horowitz, including some wonderful sonatas by Scar-
latti. Erica also has other CDs, not many, half a dozen,
but tonight the "Heroic" Polonaise is enough for us, all the
music in the world is summed up in the "Heroic" Polonaise,
which in Horowitz's interpretation lasts six minutes and
fifteen seconds and which we must have listened to fifteen
or twenty times in succession. We continued to dance to
the strains of this music, which is anything but danceable,
writhing in joy and ecstasy when the piano leaps up to the
stars and when, without losing momentum, it allows itself
the intoxication of slowing down, and in such a state of
shared euphoria the question of sleeping together was necessarily on the table. Very wisely we didn't, though I no
longer remember just how and thanks to whom this mistake was avoided. No matter: in a way, Erica and I made
love that night.

Locked in

I wake up at 3 a.m., my throat dry, my head on fire, consumed with anxiety and knowing that I'll pay dearly for that moment of euphoria. I go to drink some water in the kitchen, several huge glasses from the tap, and search in vain for an aspirin in the medicine cabinet. Fortunately there's a toilet on the ground floor, which I use, but the only washroom is upstairs, next to Erica's room, in fact *in* Erica's room, and I think that I really have to get out of here and find a room in town—which in the end I never did. Certain that I won't go back to sleep, I decide to go for a walk outside and wander through the deserted streets. I like to walk at random, as randomly as possible, trying to get lost, but the truth is that it's not easy to get lost in a village like this where, even when you turn your back on the sea, after ten minutes you inevitably end up at the port. But when I try to open the front door a surprise awaits me: it's locked. From the inside, with a key that someone has removed—that "someone" being necessarily Erica. Why? Even a lonely, slightly paranoid woman who's used to locking the door before going to bed will leave the key in the lock. There are only two windows on the ground floor, the one in my room and the one in the kitchen, and they both have bars, which I found quite creepy when I arrived. Did Erica take the key with her to her room? Did she deliberately lock me in? I waver between anger, thoughts about the blame I'll heap on her in a few hours' time, and detached curiosity about such incomprehensible behavior. What should I do until morning? I don't have the courage for yoga or meditation. I didn't bring any books with me but there are about fifteen on a shelf, and I look them over. Unlike Erica's CDs, which truly reflect her taste that's so much like mine, these books say nothing about her. They must have been there when she moved in: an odd array of paperbacks in several languages, a Tom Clancy spy thriller, the relational self-help book *Men Are from Mars, Women Are from Venus*, an out-of-date Lonely Planet travel guide, not even about Greece but about the Sultanate of Oman . . . Ah! What could be hers is a manual on mindfulness meditation . . . Then at the far end of the shelf another surprise awaits me, and a big one at that: a well-worn edition, in English, of George Langelaan's short stories called *Out of Time*. I read this book when I was a teenager, and I've never forgotten it. The French edition was published by Marabout, a cheap collection of fantasy and science-fiction novels, whose catalogue I can still recite by heart today. Nothing has played a greater role in shaping my tastes than these stories. On the last page of this book there's a photo and a brief biographical note that leaves you thinking. Apart from his very occasional work as a fiction writer, George Langelaan was a British liaison officer for the French resistance during the Second World War. He even went so far as having facial surgery before being parachuted into occupied France so as to look the part of a French collaborator—or at least of someone's idea of what a French collaborator should look like. The photo shows a small, pudgy, sour-faced, slightly daft-looking man, and you can't help wondering what George Langelaan looked like before he sacrificed what could well have been a better physique in the interests of Free France. Knowing this biographical trait, it's somewhat disturbing that his most famous story, "The Fly," describes the tragic metamorphosis of a scientist who attempts a daring experiment in teleportation. Only unlike Bismillah from Tiruvannamalai, he doesn't rely solely on the powers of the mind and Vipassana meditation, but on the typical accoutrements of 1950s sci-fi, the idea being to lock himself in a cabinet bristling with electrodes, to vanish and reconstitute himself identically, cell for cell, in another cabinet bristling with electrodes at the other end of the lab. The first experiments are encouraging, but disaster strikes in the form of a fly that he inadvertently locks in the cabinet with him, so that what is disintegrated and then reconstituted cell for cell is not just him, but a frightening mixture of *him and the fly*. This memorable short story has been adapted for the cinema twice, the more deservedly famous version being, as I've said, the one by David Cronenberg, which is not only

terrifying but also heartbreaking. But all of this is a bit
beside the point, because that night I don't read "The Fly"
but another short story, "Recession," which I'd vowed to
reread after my Vipassana retreat. But then came *Charlie
Hebdo* and my own personal meltdown, and my vow has
all but slipped my mind until I find myself at the home
of this music-loving medievalist from Boise, Idaho, who,
by locking me in her damp, gloomy house, has given me
the gift of these twenty pages, which, although I've barely
glanced at them in the past forty-five years, I realize I still
know almost by heart.

George Langelaan's short story

An old man is dying. Doctors and nurses in white coats
busy themselves around his bed. Instruments clink on a
metal tray. A needle is stuck into his arm. Muffled voices
sound like the ones he used to hear when he was a tod-
dler falling asleep in his mother's arms. A tube is slipped
into his mouth. A sound of metal clanking, and then he's
pushed on a stretcher down a very long, narrow, dark corridor. A light shines high above his head. Lying down as he
is, he can see it clearly. He hears the voice of his eldest son:
"Is he still conscious?" "Not really. He's already far gone . . ."
The corridor has become even narrower, the light above him
even more distant. Then the voices fade away. Suddenly he
realizes that he can no longer see anything, hear anything,
or feel anything. He's in the dark. Will someone come?
Will someone turn the light back on? Is anyone still there?

Are his son and the others still standing around him, looking into his waxy face and wondering if behind it, distant
and out of reach, he's still conscious at all? He tries to
lift an eyelid, but he can't. To scream, but he can't hear
himself. Who will hear him if he can't hear himself? Is
he in a coma? Or: *Is he dead?* Is what's happening to him
now not simply death? No sooner has he thought this than
he knows the answer: yes, that's it. It's death. "I'm dead."
But at the same time, if he can think he's dead, it means
that his brain is still functioning, his blood is still flowing,
his heart hasn't stopped beating. Then it strikes him that
what remains conscious in him, the thing that can say "I'm
dead," that can say "I," is his soul—the part of him that
cannot perish. Has he already been buried? No sensations,
no way of knowing. No way of situating himself in space, no
way of measuring time. It's terrifying. The most terrifying
thing is that he's still conscious. If only he could lose consciousness! If only everything could be turned off. If only
he could at least sleep. He tries counting sheep. Calmly,
unhurriedly, more sheep than Australia will ever have. He
counts, and counts, and counts, and at one point realizes
that he's reached 998 million. 998 million sheep that he's
visualized and counted one by one, jumping over a fence in
a sunny meadow. Assuming that you can count one sheep
per second, which seems reasonable, that's 60 sheep per
minute, 3,600 per hour, 86,400 sheep per day, so it would
take twelve days of counting to get to a million sheep, and
to get almost to a billion, the figure he's reached, it would
take around twelve thousand days, so roughly thirty years.
He thought he'd been at it for half an hour, but he's been

counting sheep for thirty years. Shit. If he doesn't want to go crazy, clearly he's got to find something to do other than counting sheep. But what? Relive his whole life? Devote eternity to an eternal autobiography? With all the time in the world to go into detail: a century to describe a fifteen-minute breakfast? Or repeat a mantra endlessly, the way the mystics do? Absorb himself in chess problems? Mentally practice the form of tai chi, with no end of time to become a grandmaster? Remember the beds he slept in, the clothes he wore, the places he lived, the contents of every drawer? Think back on all the times he made love? And with whom? And which positions followed which? Spend eternity masturbating without a penis, without a body, without sensations? Strange, to be dead and still be aware of himself. Prisoner of the most perfect prison: when you're no longer anything but an awareness, you can't dig a tunnel to escape. What is possible, however, is to *imagine* that you're digging tunnels. So he starts. He decides to dig, all alone, mentally, from the bottom of his grave if—as he thinks—he's indeed buried, a tunnel that will link France and England under the English Channel. He starts by drawing up the plans. Then he builds, then he fails, then he starts again from scratch because he forgot to take the tidal range into account. He doesn't skip any steps; if a task requires ten workers, he'll be each one in turn. He's the diver whose oxygen hose breaks, and the frogman who saves the diver from drowning. He's everyone, he's everywhere, he has time to spare. In not even a few thousand years, the tunnel is finished. It's more constructive, and more satisfying, than counting billions and billions of sheep. On the strength of this experience, he sets about building a completely new city, bigger than Brasília. Every building, every concrete block, every door handle, every switch, the electrical system controlling every switch: nothing is missing. And even if it's all in his mind, it all works. Why not aim even higher, then? Why not create life? How do you create life? There aren't fifty thousand solutions: by creating a cell. Although he knows even less about embryology than he does about architecture, he can't delegate anything to imaginary workers and must do everything himself. All he knows is that one cell divides into two cells, which then divide in turn, until a mountain of cells turns into something you can see under a microscope. But it's not easy to change yourself into a cell when what you're reduced to, what you can still call yourself, is infinitely smaller and more immaterial than a cell. You have to concentrate on becoming a billion times bigger. He concentrates. He puts his entire consciousness into a point that gradually grows and becomes a cell, which divides into two cells, which divide in turn, until this group of cells becomes something like a rudimentary body, something that can move in space and experience sensations. He feels what an astronaut must feel when he touches down after a long interstellar journey. He touches down. He lands. He didn't burn up, he's not dead, he's happy. He has no mouth to laugh or shout for joy with, not yet. And suddenly he does, he becomes aware that he has one—an opening, a slit that will become a mouth with teeth, a tongue. His consciousness now inhabits a brain, made of cells and extended in a still shapeless mass, a sort of sack that will soon have limbs, organs, a sex, an asshole, and all of this will be *him*. Now he can go to sleep. He sleeps at last, a perfect, blissful sleep. There's nothing better than this sleep, nothing better than bathing in the soft warmth of amniotic fluid. He's an embryo, soon he'll be a body that diligently continues to change and grow. The body of whom, the body of what? He still has no idea, but no matter: whatever it is, he'll live the life he's been given. If he has to be born an ant, fine, he'll be an ant, any life will do. He has no desire to leave samsara, all he wants is to live again. And he's lucky: he's a fetus, soon to be a baby human, already kicking his feet. Then comes the terrifying moment when the warm, liquid environment in which he was peacefully dozing suddenly empties: it's like being in a sinking submarine. He chokes, but doesn't drown. He enters a dark, hot, slippery tunnel. He can't breathe: no wonder so many people relive this in their nightmares. He hears noise, voices. The noises and voices that faded when he died are getting closer now. Or rather, he's getting closer. The tunnel becomes a slide. He slides. A great flash of light blinds him. It's the exit. His mother pushes, his mother screams. He's arrived. He's the one who's screaming now. His life begins.

Molecular yoga

When my grandson Louis was born, I read this story, which so impressed me when I was thirteen or fourteen and which still impresses me no end, to my daughter Jeanne. It filled her with wonder—especially the end, when she suddenly

understood what it was about. At the hospital, she looked
for a trace of this odyssey in her nephew's eyes. A blurred
look, the look of a newborn baby who understands nothing
but is already starting to adapt. And also, barely visible, the
look of a very old man who for a few moments still remembers where he came from. I think about it sometimes, when
I'm meditating. I thought about it during the Vipassana retreat. It's another definition of meditation, the thirteenth:
digging tunnels, building dams, opening lanes, bringing
something into being in the infinite space that opens up inside you. Advanced meditators must be able to create such
construction sites, while the rest of us can at best only see
the fencing around them. This reminds me of something
the great Iyengar yoga master Faek Biria told us during a
class on basic postures. They all seemed quite easy, but he
got us to hold them for a very long time. To help us through
what turned out to be an exhausting session, he told us
stories. Slowly, calmly, like a Persian storyteller: here his
Iranian culture really came to the fore. At one point he
told us that when you start practicing these simple postures it's at the level of the bones, then of the muscles,
then of the joints. That's more or less where we were at,
he said. And, provided we didn't give up, at one point we'd
reach the cellular, and even the molecular level. Yes: *cellular, molecular*. Through yoga, Faek said quietly, you can fill
each of your cells, each of your molecules, with awareness.
You can get to know each one, personally. You can control
each one, personally. We had a good laugh about that after the class, over bulgur salad and Swiss chard pies under
a huge plane tree, each of us nonchalantly trying to pick

out the softest peaches, but I'm sure Faek wasn't joking. I'll never get there, but I think you can practice yoga, the same yoga postures, at the cellular and molecular levels. By paying attention to your skin and what's under your skin, to your inhalation and your exhalation, to the pumping of your heart, the circulation of your blood, and the ebb and flow of your thoughts, by diving into this infinitely tenuous pool of sensations and consciousness, I'm sure that one day you'll come out on the other side, into an infinitely great, infinitely open space, into the sky that man was born to contemplate: that's yoga.

The Samsung Galaxy

Laurence, the journalist friend through whom I met Erica, had said I should bring some small presents for the young refugees I'd meet on Leros. Apart from money, which she didn't recommend, the most welcome gifts are Vodafone refill cards. I've never used such cards, and rather than buying what might not be the right kind, I resolved to go with the boys themselves so they could choose their own. But now, dunking a Lipton tea bag in my bowl, I have another idea, a gift for the neediest of our little group, Hassan. I can't get someone to help him pack his bag the night before he left, but there is another way I can help to alleviate his misfortune: I can give him a smartphone, since he's the only one without one. This plan obviously raises some questions: Why give such an expensive gift just to him? What will the others think? I'm aware of these objections but I dismiss them out of hand, the way you do when you're

seized by the compulsive need to buy and nothing seems
more necessary or urgent than snapping up a high-end Bluetooth speaker or the writings of the Pre-Socratic philoso-
phers in the leather-bound, gold-stamped Pleiades edition.
This morning I want to buy a smartphone for Hassan, my
only concern being that maybe you can't get one on the island, and I'm relieved to find a small phone shop in the port.
Not an Apple Store, of course, but I'm not planning on buying him an iPhone anyway. None of the boys have one, that
would be a provocation. I choose a Samsung Galaxy for
240 euros, without knowing exactly how to use it, I mean
whether you have to take out a subscription with a service
provider or if Vodafone cards will suffice. As we walk up
the now familiar road to the Pikpa, I worry about how I'm
going to give it to him. In fact there are only two ways,
either openly or in secret, and both of them are bad. I'm
not about to lure Hassan into a corner, hand him the little
bundle like a drug dealer, and let him say it fell from the
sky. But I'm not going to get everyone together and pretend
it's his birthday either—though all things considered that
might not be as bad as the first option, as the boys seem to
have a strong sense of solidarity. I haven't yet made up my
mind when we arrive and Hamid tells us that Hassan has
left. Not gone for a walk or skipped class: really left. Disappeared. His bed is made, his bag is missing and so are
his things. Hamid's the only one who speaks. Mohamed's
silence is normal, but Atiq's isn't, and I understand that he
blames himself for provoking Hassan's departure by theat-
rically underscoring his misfortune the day before. Before
that Hassan was quiet, Erica tells me, shy but quiet, she's .

never seen him cry. Where can he be? Still on the island, or already on his way to Athens after slipping onto a ferry, as many of them do? And what will happen to him in Athens? Generally stowaways end up in prison, or they're sent back to the big Moria refugee camp on Lesbos. In any case they stand very little chance of getting to one of the Northern European countries they all dream of reaching. The atmosphere in the class was leaden after that. Erica gets the idea of flipping through her huge notebook for Hassan's only contribution. He recited it in Farsi, Atiq translated, and she wrote it all down. Entitled "A Journey of Hope but Full of Challenges," it's the story of his trip from Turkey to Greece. Leaving Istanbul, where he paid a fortune for a life jacket he was told he had to have, he traveled down the Turkish coast to Bodrum in the back of a van along with twenty other Afghans. There they waited for three days in a forest with hardly any food. Then, on the third night, the two smugglers took them to the beach where the boat was waiting—an old Zodiac, much smaller and more heavily laden than Hassan expected. He knows that even if the passage is short, it's the most dangerous part of the journey and the risk of drowning is high, but he has no choice. Then he sees that the life jacket he was forced to buy for half his money has a hole in it. But he can't keep it anyway, because when they get on the boat, the smugglers force them to leave everything but the clothes they're wearing on the beach. Everything, even the bags they packed in three layers of rubbish bags in Istanbul in preparation for the crossing. They have to abandon their only possessions, their most precious things. For Hassan it's a photo of his dead parents, his parents who would at least have helped him pack his bag if they'd still been alive, and he begins to cry, thinking that he'll forget their faces, that he'll soon forget everyone who knew him, everyone for whom he existed, and that soon he'll no longer exist for anyone. Erica is silent, the text stops there, the mood has sunk through the floor. We hadn't planned to say a prayer for Hassan, but of course that's what we did.

The shadow

Back at the house, I throw the Samsung Galaxy into the drawer of the bedside table, the only piece of furniture in my room besides the bed. That evening Erica and I meet for dinner and, like an old couple, we do exactly what we did the night before, except that the night before it was joyful and effusive and tonight it's stifled and laborious. Our hangovers push us as far as the sad half measure of not drinking too much. When we get back to her viewless terrace after the restaurant, for herbal tea that tastes of dust and the bottom of a cupboard, Erica has the tact not to put on the "Heroic" Polonaise, and not to play any music at all. But we do talk a bit. I ask her if the meditation manual I saw the night before on the living room shelf is hers. Yes, it is, she says. She didn't discover it through yoga—Ashtanga practitioners aren't usually wild about meditation—but following a stroke she'd had two years earlier, just after she retired and was looking forward to happy days with the Dutch bass player that never materialized. She'd come to Amsterdam to be with him, but she found herself alone in a hospital where he only came to see her infrequently, was always in a hurry, treated her stroke like no more than a bad cold, and blamed her for coddling herself. Then a few days after she got out, he told her that in addition to his wife, whom he'd always presented as a surmountable obstacle, he also had a long-standing lover for whom he still cared a lot. From then on things went from bad to worse, but in her misfortune Erica can at least be happy that she doesn't suffer from any aftereffects of her stroke. Except for one very strange carryover, which is more creepy or spooky than disabling, as she says, and very difficult to describe. It's as if behind her, on her left, there's a shapeless, dark, menacing thing, something like a bear, a black bag, thick smoke, a cloud of wasps, something indistinct, menacing and vaguely unclean, that swarms and crawls and swells and scares her. She doesn't talk about it to anyone, also because there's no one she can talk about it with. She calls it the shadow. The shadow accompanies her everywhere, and is forever springing up on her left at the edge of her field of vision. Erica spends her time watching for it out of the corner of her eye. She hopes to surprise it one day, to be faster than it, but in fact she's never been able to catch a glimpse of it. She's always *on the verge* of seeing it, as she says. In the neurological ward of the hospital in Amsterdam, where she was very well treated, she insists, a doctor taught her a meditation technique called mindfulness, saying it could

help her. Apart from its claim to be strictly scientific and
its refusal of unnecessary protocol, mindfulness meditation is in no way different from Buddhist meditation of the
Vipassana type. You sit silent and motionless, pay attention
to your breathing, and are open to everything that crosses the
field of consciousness, observing without judging, expecting nothing, letting things happen, letting go. The virtues
of this method for relieving stress are proven, it's increasingly practiced in the medical field, and there's nothing but
good to say about it. Erica left the hospital with a book
by its promoter, the American psychiatrist Jon Kabat-Zinn,
and a CD of guided meditations that she tries to listen to
regularly. "Does it make you feel good?" I ask. She says yes.
There's a pause. She says yes again, less confidently than
the last time, shakes her head as if to say no, and whereas
until now she's spoken very calmly, tears now come to her
eyes, her broad shoulders are shaken by a sort of convul-
sion, and she whispers: "Emmanuel, it's horrible . . . It's
horrible . . . It's horrible . . ." We sit opposite each other
on white plastic garden chairs, exactly like the one on the
embankment at the Vipassana retreat, and she repeats, "It's
horrible." She sobs, I lean toward her and take one of her
hands in mine, I say it's okay, it's okay. I'd like to wrap
my arms around her and comfort her like we comforted
Hassan the day before. She lifts her head, looks at me,
and says: "This meditation CD is good. And it does give
me some relief. But you see, there's lake meditation, there's
sky meditation, there's mountain meditation. You have to
imagine that your consciousness is a calm, mirror-smooth

lake, and that from time to time there are small ripples on its surface, or that there are clouds or birds passing in the sky, and you have to say to yourself that your thoughts and sensations are like these ripples or clouds or birds, you have to watch them go by without following them, without getting attached to them, you have to stay focused on the lake, or on the sky, or on the mountain, which is so solid and unshakable. And if you do it every day, they say you'll become as solid and unshakable as the mountain and at the same time full of gentleness and compassion and indulgence for your shitty thoughts and your shitty life and your shitty home on this shitty island, and that asshole who fucked up your life, and especially for the shadow . . . The shadow, Emmanuel . . . What should I do with it? You can't imagine how horrible it is, this shadow that I can't see and is always there. It's so horrible . . ." I listen to Erica, I understand what she's saying very well, terribly well. My own shadow is a pretty Raoul Dufy seascape, and it's as horrible as hers. Everyone must have one, only for most people it remains a little more discreetly behind their backs, whereas for others like us it's more directly threatening: "The magnificent and lamentable family of the nervous," Proust called us, adding that we're the salt of the earth, we the nervous, the melancholic, the bipolar, who spend our lives fighting the "black dog" of which another great depressive, Winston Churchill, spoke. I'd like to console Erica by sharing with her these words that console me a little, or by reciting to her this poem by Catherine Pozzi, which is a sort of homage to Louise Labé, and whose last lines I love so much:

Je ne sais pas pourquoi je meurs et noie
Avant d'entrer à l'éternel séjour
Je ne sais pas de qui je suis la proie
Je ne sais pas de qui je suis l'amour.

But how to translate them?

Atiq travels

An only child, Atiq lived in Afghanistan until he was two. His parents were both killed in a car accident, he tells me, and he was taken in by his aunt in Quetta, Pakistan, where she lives with her husband. The family belongs to the Hazara ethnic group, and as I know nothing about the Hazaras, he shows me the Wikipedia entry on his mobile phone. Persecuted in Afghanistan by the Taliban, they're also persecuted in Pakistan, where they've taken refuge in large numbers. Atiq's mobile phone is almost the same model as the one I wanted to give Hassan, he pays ten euros a month for 3G because he has to be connected 24/7. We're sitting by the sea in the comfortable rattan armchairs of Café Pushkin, five minutes from the Pikpa. This café, where I've started coming regularly, owes its incongruous name to Svetlana Sergeyevna, the kind Russian lady who's been running it for more than twenty years. Svetlana has covered all the walls with icons, she crosses herself nonstop, and drinks her tea, as Russians do, with a lump of sugar in her mouth—I know this because we drink a glass of tea together from time to time. We talk in Russian, which makes us both happy. Scooters pass by, backfiring on the dusty road. When I show surprise that Atiq drinks beer, he shrugs and says that Islam tolerates certain freedoms when you're traveling: you don't have to pray five times a day, for example. So we drink a couple of bottles of the Greek beer Mythos, only somehow I manage to spill a bottle, smudging and rendering almost unreadable the Google Maps image of the Middle East that I've printed out to follow his story. Atiq's aunt's husband owns a three-story department store, the top floor of which also serves as a wedding hall. They have two sons and a daughter, Parwana, who in the photo Atiq shows me exudes grace, gentleness, and joy. Each of them has a room in the flat above the department store, and Atiq has never been treated as a second-class relative. He's also protected by his uncle, who's a cook in Brussels and whom he's seen only once in person, when he was little, but with whom he talks once a week on Skype. His uncle sends him money, which he uses to buy a new motorbike each year. He shows me a photo of himself on the latest one, a Yamaha 150. He looks like a happy, carefree teenager. It was while he was riding this bike that he was shot. Who shot him? Why was he shot? Was it personal, revenge against his family, or was he just unlucky enough to be in the wrong place at the wrong time? He doesn't know, and neither does anyone in his family, apparently. Two bystanders were killed, he was hit in the shoulder.

He unbuttons his shirt to show me the scar. When he
hears what's happened, his uncle the cook in Brussels decides that things are getting out of hand in Quetta, and
starts saying that it's time for Atiq to leave. After a lot of
talk in which Atiq is not involved, we come to the scene he
described in his assignment. The second time I hear it I
wonder: If Quetta has become so dangerous and you risk
being shot at every corner, especially if you're Hazara, why
is Atiq the only one who has the privilege to leave? Why
not his cousins? Why not Parwana? First, he tells me as a
matter of course, the trip is very dangerous, so it's both a
privilege and not a privilege. And second, he's the only one
with a relative abroad who's willing to take him in and pay
four thousand dollars for the trip. His uncle had to pay the
smugglers in two installments: two thousand for the trip
from Quetta to Tehran, and the same amount from Tehran
to Greece. As for Atiq, he leaves with two hundred dollars
in his pocket. The sports bag his aunt helped him pack
contains two pairs of jeans, two T-shirts, four pairs of un-
derwear, a fleece jacket, a toiletry kit, four half-liter bottles
of water, a carton of Player's cigarettes, headphones, and in
a frame, a picture of his parents with him as a baby in his
mother's arms. Atiq likes motorbikes and cars, he remembers that the car that came to pick him up was a Toyota
Corolla XLI. It arrived at four in the morning, his aunt and
her husband went down to the front entrance with him, he
kissed them and got in the back, where there was only one
other passenger, a guy around thirty-five. The windows of
the car were tinted, so he could still see his relatives but
they couldn't see him. They waved to him but not quite in

the right direction, then the car pulled out. Atiq didn't talk at all with his traveling companion, who didn't seem interested in talking either. He felt bad, he couldn't decide if he was grateful to his uncle or angry with him for dragging him on this trip. He thought that if his parents hadn't died, he wouldn't be there. Atiq shows me the first stages of his journey on the map, which has almost dried by now. First they drive all day through a landscape of cracked ocher mud. When night falls, the driver leaves him and his companion in front of an abandoned warehouse and tells them to wait, they'll be picked up. Atiq asks when, the driver shrugs. The warehouse is situated on the outskirts of a city. They have no idea which city it could be. At the time Atiq thought it might be Kandahar, but looking at the map today he's no longer sure. There can be no question of exploring the surrounding area, they could miss the next ride. The two have little choice but to exchange a few words. The other man is also Hazara; that helps to break the ice. He wants to go to Germany, where his two brothers live. He offers Atiq a cereal bar. In the immediate vicinity there's nothing more comfortable to sleep on than the cold floor of the warehouse, and they decide to take turns. The other guy has a coat and a sweater. Atiq shivers, and begins to suspect that the cold is going to be a problem. He doesn't understand why his family gave him so few warm clothes. In the middle of the night, they're awakened by headlights and the screeching of a pickup truck. A guy gets out and tells them to get in. Get in where? There are already four men sitting in the most coveted seats, in the front next to the driver. When they lift the tarp and look in

the back, they discover thirty or so people squeezed together like battery hens. Not a gap, nowhere to squeeze in.
The situation is clear: you push, you push, you can always
make a little more room by pushing a little more, but then
a critical point comes when you can't push anymore. No
matter how hard you try, you can't squeeze anymore and
you have to face the facts: there's no more room. That's
what a woman sitting near the exit with a baby in her arms
lets them know with an apologetic smile. Atiq and his
companion stand at a loss beside the pickup waiting for
someone to find a solution, but neither the driver nor his
helper seem to be looking for one. The engine is running,
the two are going to be left behind, so they grab on to the
back of the pickup. For at least sixty miles they either stand
on the rear fender and cling to the metal uprights, or they
sit on the rim of the tailgate, which cuts into their buttocks
and legs. Either way they risk falling at any moment. Later
in the trip, Atiq will witness such an accident on another
pickup, as the pickups will be changed several times. The
next time he's managed to find a place in the chicken coop.
He's suffocating, but he can doze off because when you're
packed together like that you hardly feel the bumps. And
you aren't cold either. Suddenly there's a shout, the driver
hits the brakes: a young guy his age who was standing on
the fender like he was has just fallen off. Then, Atiq says,
looking me squarely in the eye in case I don't believe him,
the driver doesn't come to a full stop, he just runs over the
boy, crushing him and continuing on his way, not caring
about the screams of an older guy who Atiq understands

must be the boy's brother. There's something I don't get about this story: in order for the driver to run over the boy, he'd have had to back up. That is, instead of stopping for a minute to pick him up, he had to spend that minute deliberately driving over him: Is that what happened? Yes, says Atiq, that's what happened. I'm still puzzled. I've made films before, and this feels like one of those sequences that you can write into a screenplay but when the time comes to shoot it, you can't because it doesn't make sense. On March 1 they reach the Iranian border. It's a mountainous barrier, impossible to cross by car, and the slope they have to climb seems almost vertical. Several pickups converge on the meeting point, and Atiq now becomes part of a group of about fifty people, including just two women. One of them is the one with a baby, whose screams everyone dreads. The two guides paid by the smugglers to lead the group are from Balochistan. They speak Balochi, which Atiq understands a little, but he doesn't speak to them. In general, he won't talk to anyone during the trip and no one will talk to him, although Atiq is nothing if not sociable. But that's how it is: when you're in the same boat with everyone else and should really be helping and reassuring one another, and when most of the time you've got nothing else to do, you don't talk. You wait, you're afraid, you stay quiet. Afterward, in Istanbul, Atiq will understand: the four thousand dollars his uncle paid is a small fee entitling him to minimal benefits and the most difficult, dangerous crossing. The richer ones cross the mountains over more comfortable paths: the more you pay, the less you climb.

Atiq, on the other hand, spends a day and a half trudging up and down hills, crossing snowfields with his skimpy running shoes and nothing more than his fleece to protect him from the cold ground on the freezing nights, whereas most of the others have parkas. What were his aunt and her husband thinking when they gave him fifty dollars to buy jeans and T-shirts, instead of saying go buy yourself a parka, the warmest one you can find, and gloves, and trekking shoes, and woolen long johns to wear under your jeans? A sleeping bag would be perfect, but no one has one because they're too bulky, and those who did have one had it confiscated at the start. Atiq layers all his clothes on top of one another, which is hardly better than nothing at all. In this way they arrive, on foot, in Saravan. Now they start to cross Iran. Atiq tries to show me the stages on the map, but soon gives up because he didn't see any of it. He spent most of the journey in the luggage compartment of a bus—well, no, he corrects himself, not in the luggage compartment: in a cache built *under* the luggage compartment where he was cooped up with eight people for forty-eight hours, locked in from the outside, lying down, unable to get out or move. At one point someone had a panic attack, it was horrible. Nevertheless, Atiq blessed that rolling coffin when they heard the police searching the hold a few inches above them, and pulling out a screaming boy whom they never saw again. It took them four days to reach Tehran, and there things were better. Atiq's uncle has a friend in Tehran, in whose apartment Atiq spent four days resting. A room, sheets, a shower whenever he wanted, meals, an outlet to charge his phone, people who talked to him nicely: he'd forgotten such things existed. He'd have liked to stay there, live in Tehran and get Parwana to come join him, why not? But that wasn't how either Atiq's uncle or Atiq's uncle's friend saw things. He left Tehran on March 9, and his story becomes even more convoluted as the vehicles change, the groups remain more or less the same but keep swelling and shrinking with each stage. They're all Afghans like him, and they all speak Farsi, but again they don't talk to one another. They travel by night, he can't see anything outside. It's very hot during the day, very cold at night, and on March 15 they get to the icy border separating Iran and Turkey, and once again they're deep in the mountains. They climb from eight at night to three in the morning, then they rest until six, but Atiq is so cold in these three hours that he thinks he'll stop there, die there. The saddest thing is that he finds the mountains beautiful: there are flowers, if there were a shelter it'd be wonderful. If he were rich, Atiq would buy a little house in the mountains, he'd build a fire in the fireplace, there'd be beds with thick quilts, you'd see the snow swirling past the windows. They start down the Turkish side, and looking at the map I realize that the nearest town to the mountain, on the edge of a lake, is called Van, and that it's in the same rough vicinity as Kars, where I've never been but which for me has enormous literary prestige because it's where Orhan Pamuk's novel *Snow* takes place. What if I went there? What if I went to Van, to Kars, to Kandahar, and to Quetta? What if I toured all these places? What if I did Atiq's trip in reverse? Even if I did it under infinitely less adventurous and dangerous conditions than Atiq did, this journey could be a return trip, like Odysseus' voyage back to Ithaca. Finally, I'd arrive at dawn in the sleeping house. I'd put down my bag, stroke the little cat we called Feta because he's white and Greek, and I'd say to myself, here I am, I've come home, and even though I know very well that it's not going to happen, that I've done absolutely everything to make sure it doesn't happen, for a few moments I let myself get caught up in this reverie, which Atiq interrupts by asking with concern: "Are you okay?" I say yes, I'm okay, I was just thinking about things in my life. "Sad things?" Atiq asks— apparently my face doesn't lie. Atiq nods, he knows about sad things, now he's got one to tell me. "A terrible thing," even. The woman with the baby, the one who's been there since the start, squished like a battery hen in the first pickup when Atiq and the other guy were trying to get in, the woman with the baby abandons her baby. It's been screaming for a while, the smuggler has been grumbling, she's been trying to calm it—you try calming a baby in such conditions. She has nothing to feed it. She has no more milk, and no one else has any either. They give the baby opium pellets to keep it quiet, but it keeps on screaming, the smuggler threatens the mother so she does what he orders: she abandons the baby. She puts it on the ground in a flat, grassy place, and keeps going with them, leaving it behind. No one picks up the baby, no one saves it, no one can help anyone, it's everyone for himself. "That was the most difficult moment of my journey," Atiq comments soberly, "I haven't stopped thinking about it. I don't know what I should do with it." I nod. What should I say? A few months later, in Paris, I tell this story to a friend who works for an NGO. He says: "You know, these guys clearly went through hell, but they were also told what to say to get political refugee status. There's a standard narrative, and in that standard narrative the baby being force-fed opium and then left to the vultures in the mountains is a required episode. I'm not saying it doesn't happen, and I'm not saying the boy you're talking about didn't actually see it happen. I'm just saying it can't happen every time." Okay. Here, too, what should I say? But I believe Atiq. We order a last round of Mythos, we're reaching the end of his trip. I'll skip the two days in Van, which is apparently no longer as sleepy as it was in the days of Orhan Pamuk's novel, but an open-air refugee camp, teeming with young migrants the way Kathmandu teems with trekkers. I'll skip the ride across Turkey on a fairly comfortable night bus with TV monitors showing music videos and wildlife films. And I'll skip Istanbul, where they stay for a week, fifteen of them crammed in a flat that's small and dirty but very close to a bazaar where they're allowed to go in turns. Atiq is now on a beach from where you can see the lights of the Bodrum marina, one of the most luxurious in Europe, with boats costing easily ten million dollars. It's on this dark beach that Atiq meets Hassan and their stories overlap. He recalls the traumatic episode when they had to abandon their bags before getting on the boat. Someone tried to protest, and the Turkish trafficker told him: "If you're not happy, don't get in. If you don't get in, I'll shoot you. And if I shoot you, no one will know." They were terrified during the crossing, they prayed, but the waves weren't too high, they were lucky, and lucky also to reach land safely after four hours. They wanted to smoke on the beach, but all their matches and lighters were soaked. Atiq tried to dry his remaining half-pack of Player's. As I'd been listening to him for more than two hours, my attention wandered and I didn't quite catch how their little group split up, how he managed to reach Lesbos, or how he ended up walking alone on a road where he was picked up by a couple of French tourists. I can imagine the impression Atiq made on them all the more because I've been in the same situation. What do you do when you're suddenly face to face with a young guy who's totally destitute, I mean who has literally nothing, who's just made an unimaginable journey under unimaginable conditions? You buy him a Coke, a sandwich, give him twenty euros, pat him on the back, and tell him he's brave and that he'll be fine. That's what I did, and that's what the French tourists did too, and they found it very hard to refuse the half-pack of wet Player's, Atiq's only possession, which he insisted on giving them in exchange for the Coke. He found Hassan and met Hamid in the Moria refugee camp, where there were three thousand people at the time. Now there are sixteen thousand whose lives and dreams have washed up there. As unaccompanied minors, Atiq, Hassan, and Hamid were transferred to Leros. Since the four thousand dollars paid by his uncle covered the Quetta–Tehran trip and then Tehran–Istanbul, Atiq assumed that once he reached Europe his journey would be over, and that he'd simply take a bus to join his uncle in Brussels. He was soon disillusioned, and now he wonders on good days when he'll arrive in Brussels, and on bad days if he'll get to Brussels at all, or if he won't be left to rot in one hot spot after the next, like an eternal beggar in front of the door to the real world, to real life. I'm so impressed by Atiq's intelligence, charm, and strength that I tell him, sincerely but also a little lightly, that I'm not worried about him: he'll be fine. Atiq nods: he's not so sure.

The bad nap

As we relax after this three-hour debriefing over a last bottle of Mythos, Atiq asks me what I plan to do with what
he's just told me. However sensible, this question leaves me
speechless. The answer is: I don't know. I don't know what to
do with it, I don't know what to do with myself, I don't know
what to do with anything. I answer vaguely: an article. When
will it come out? He expects it to be by the end of the week,
and more on an online platform than in a newspaper. I'm
evasive: I need more time. Today, Atiq has surely forgotten
the haggard man in the dirty shirt with the trembling hands
whom he hung out with when he first arrived in Europe, and
he'd certainly be very surprised to learn that this interview
in Café Pushkin about his perilous journey from Pakistan to
Greece has resurfaced, four years later, in something as unlikely as a book on yoga—well, in something that was supposed to be a book on yoga, and after many metamorphoses

may actually turn out to be one. In the meantime, Atiq feels a bit like he's been tricked. Erica, meanwhile, is worried about an email she's just received from a humanitarian association that's concerned about her methods: Shouldn't she be consulting a psychologist about her writing workshop? Shouldn't she be following proven protocols? And the fact is, the kind of wild therapy to which we're subjecting the boys disturbs them. More and more often when we arrive at the Pikpa, we find them deep in a lethargic nap, and we have the hardest time persuading them to get up, sit down at the tables, and open their notebooks. Hamid is exactly the way he describes himself in his post: always smiling, but behind that smile totally defeated, lost. As for Atiq, whom we have to get out of the shower, where he spends as much time as possible, he says he doesn't want to talk about the past anymore because it hurts too much. By the past he means his mostly happy years as a child and teenager in Quetta. Erica tells him that he's not obliged to do anything, he can stop whenever he wants, it's entirely up to him, and despite his obvious affection for her he suddenly looks furious. At a loss, Erica and I hold session at Café Pushkin. One of the causes of this crisis, she says, is the imbalance between our situations. We make them tell their stories, but we don't tell them any of our own. It's too unequal a deal.

Kotelnich

Fifteen years ago, I made a documentary film in a Russian town called Kotelnich. The shooting took place over several

months, during which time my small team and I met a
lot of people, the most interesting of whom—those who
would go from being townspeople to characters—were the
local police chief and his young wife. He, Sasha, was handsome, charming, but also corrupt, alcoholic, paranoid. One
day he'd put every possible obstacle in our way, the next
he'd lavish us—Russian-style—with declarations of eternal friendship. She, Anya, was pretty, dreamy, with a tendency to exaggerate, if not lie. She adored all things French
and was spellbound by our presence, as if we were—as
she put it—the magi. We were intrigued by them, we
liked them. Then something terrible happened: Anya was
murdered, butchered with an ax by a madman, together
with her eight-month-old baby. Rumor had it that Sasha
had something to do with it. We filmed the mourning, the
funeral meal, the family's grief and heartbreak. The more
we filmed them, the more we became part of this family.
Back in Paris, I started editing and, as I went on, I spotted
connections between what we'd experienced in Kotelnich
and, in my own life, one of those painful things known as a
family secret, which can haunt several generations. At the
cost of many tears and transgressions, I gave a semblance
of burial to a dead man, my maternal grandfather, whom
no one had been able to bury or mourn, and who had become a ghost. I intertwined these two stories: theirs, mine.
Their family, my family, our tragedies. When the editing
was finished, I returned to Kotelnich to show the film to
the people who had become its actors, first and foremost
Sasha. I was nervous about how he'd react. Together we
watched the videocassette I'd brought on his TV, which

was so old that I was surprised to see the images in color. At the end, Sasha stared at me for a long time in silence, and finally said: "That's good. You didn't just come to take our pain: you brought your own as well."

An experience of departure and loss

Never has a compliment on my work touched me so much. Although I tend to think of myself as a bad man, never in my life have I felt so much like a—well, maybe not a good man, but at least a just one. I tell this to Erica in the evening on the terrace, where our conversations have taken on a much more confident, intimate tone than those at the Pikpa or Café Pushkin. I go into more detail about what you've just read. In fact, I tell her the whole film, scene by scene, reciting the dialogue almost by heart. This account lasts as long as the film itself—if I didn't rein myself in it'd last even longer, like the tai chi form when you decide to perform it slower than usual. I'm happy to do it, as it takes my mind off my own distress, and Erica proves to be a very good audience. "That's it!" she shouts at the end. "That's the way to do it! What we have to do," she goes on, "is tell our own experiences of departure and loss, a moment when our own lives were turned upside down." Erica's enthusiasm makes me uncomfortable. What story could I tell? An experience of departure and loss, a moment when my life is turned upside down, is exactly what I'm going through right now. But how can I tell our students that I'm doing it to myself? I've often repeated that you have to respect your own suffering and not play it down, and that neurotic unhappiness is no less cruel than ordinary unhappiness, but still: compared with the upheavals these sixteen- or seventeen-year-old boys have gone through and are still going through, someone who has absolutely everything it takes to be happy and who manages to ruin this happiness, as well as that of his family, is an obscenity that I can't see myself asking them to understand, and it proves my parents right when they say that during the war people didn't really have the time to be neurotic.

Fast and slow

Erica has no such reservations. She gets caught up in the game. The project of relating something important she's been through in a few pages, ten minutes of reading, to make the boys understand that she, too, has experienced hardship, becomes a sort of self-analysis in the days that follow. She works on it in the morning, filling the pages of a large notebook, identical to the one she opens and puts on the table at the beginning of our workshops, except that this one is entirely dedicated to her. One notebook for the others, one for her: I agree, you gain nothing by forgetting yourself. Evening after evening during our conversations on the terrace, washed down with our usual cheap white plonk, she reads or tells me parts of it, the way I told her my film. I listen to her with friendship and interest—even if I get a little lost in the long, sad litany of the men she's loved and who've all disappointed and disdained her, right down to the last one, the Dutch bass player for whom she left everything, after which this intelligent, generous, and decent woman was left with nothing and nobody on earth. Apart from a sister she doesn't even know is alive and a son who lives in Australia and whom she hasn't seen for years, she's totally alone. If she falls sick tomorrow, no one will take care of her. To fill this void, ever since she ran aground on Leros, there are the boys on whom she heaps an affection that's both delicate and all-consuming. And now there's me, whom she's kept locked in her house since day one—a slightly alarming *acte manqué*. I'm Erica's sparring partner, co-scriptwriter, literary adviser. She should avoid telling the boys too much about her hard-luck love affairs, I suggest as cautiously as I can, because they come from cultures that are both prudish and macho and may look down on her because of them. Erica agrees, but my advice brings her down. What should she say, then? Then the idea strikes her as a matter of course, the most surprising thing being that in the three days of our sort-of-writing workshop it hasn't struck her already. She can tell the story of her separation from her sister. This sister, Claire, is schizophrenic. Here Erica hesitates between "she is" and "she was." Her sister's psychiatric problems began early. And while Erica was a brilliant student from kindergarten on, Claire was never able to go to school. She spent long periods lying prostrate on her bed, alternated with brief moments of agitation that the whole family dreaded because she could become violent. With them, but more often with herself. One time she locked herself in a closet with an ax and tried to cut her arm off. The only thing that could calm her down was music. She'd started playing the piano as a child and, although she stopped taking lessons early on, she continued to play all her life, almost every day. She was good, Erica said, she knew a lot of pieces by heart. What she really loved were ones that demanded a high level of virtuosity, her favorite being Chopin's "Heroic" Polonaise. I looked up, Erica nodded: "Yes. You know, listening to it with you was a huge sign of trust. Normally I listen to it alone." "She could *really* play it?" I asked, surprised. "Yes, she could really play it. She made mistakes, but she played fast, very fast, faster than the indicated tempo. That's what she loved, playing the piece as fast as possible. So she rehearsed and rehearsed, she must have worked on it several hours a day for years, with a stopwatch. All the great pianists play it in around seven minutes: Rubinstein, Pollini, Arrau, Gilels, I've listened to them all, compared them all. The fastest is Horowitz, six minutes fifteen. I'm not sure he's right to play it so fast, it seems that Chopin hated it when it was played too fast, but still, it's his version I prefer because he plays it more like Claire did—well, you know what I mean. She once managed to play it in five minutes forty." I asked: "She didn't also try to play it *as slowly* as possible by any chance, did she?" "No: only very fast. It was in everyday life that she went very slowly. Her whole life took place in slow motion. Moving a spoon from her plate to her mouth could take five minutes, and in those five minutes there was no way to reach her. But when you listened to her play, you were with her. It was the only way you could really be with her. And then our parents died in a car accident." "Together? Like Atiq's?" "Yes, like

Atiq's. I lived in Boise, they lived with Claire in Kansas City. We didn't know what to do with her, so we found a foster home with some good people who had a piano. I went to see her once a month. I visited her three times like that. Each time I found her more withdrawn, more silent. She didn't see me. She was getting slower and slower: now it took her half an eternity to move the spoon from the plate to her mouth. Sometimes it seemed as if she were completely still, with the spoon hanging in the air first at one height, then at another. One day I spent the whole afternoon watching her, and I realized that this afternoon, these four or five hours, was the time she needed to make this movement, to cover the foot or so between her plate and her mouth. I wondered if she'd slow down even more. If a time would come when such a simple gesture would take her a whole day, and after that, why not more? Then she stopped playing the piano. The slowness took her away, drew her in like an abyss. The last time I went there, I left thinking that even though her foster parents were good people, I'd have to find another solution. I didn't know that that was the last time I'd see her. The next day they called and said she'd disappeared. And you know, Emmanuel, we never found her. We never did. We did all the searches we could, we never found her. When an obese, forty-five-year-old woman who never leaves the house goes out the door, she shouldn't be able to get very far. Normally you should be able to find her in a few minutes. Well, no. No one has the slightest idea what could have happened to her. That's it. That was sixteen years ago." I ask, "Was she your younger sister or your older sister?" "We're the same age,"

Erica replies matter-of-factly. "We're twins." I'm stunned: "Really? You're twins? You never told me that . . ." Erica makes a vague, slightly annoyed gesture, as if it were an insignificant detail that had no bearing on her story: "Yes, we're twins," she says, the way she might say: "Yes, we both liked gardening." And then she asks me anxiously: "Do you think it's a good story of departure and loss? Do you think they'll like it?" I reply that I'm not sure our boys like such sad stories, and that people who have very difficult lives often prefer happy stories and happy endings, but that it blew me away. The next day at the Pikpa we start with some harmless exercises, more grammar than narration, then Erica begins. Her voice trembles a little but her tic has subsided, she's stopped looking over her left shoulder for the shadow. "Now it's my turn to tell you my story," she says. "A story I've never told anyone because I never felt anyone was ready to hear it. Except you. But maybe it's not the right time. What do you think?" The question is rhetorical, but Hamid, with his usual smile hiding his tears, answers softly, "No, it's not the right time."

A night on the town

Three days after telling me the story of her twin sister, Erica says in passing, as if she were talking about going out shopping, that she's decided to leave for Brisbane, Australia. That's where her son lives, she hasn't seen him for ten years. She's counting on me to run the workshop and live in the house in her absence. Saying no is out of the question. She spends a lot of time upstairs in her room, no doubt packing her bags. And she decides to organize a party with the boys to celebrate her departure. Together we'll go down with her to the ferry pier. I wish I'd thought of it first: when you're lonely, it's nicer to have your friends hold a party for you than when you have to organize it yourself. Although I'm anything but a tightwad, I lack imagination when it comes to generosity, especially at the moment. Not counting the Samsung Galaxy that's still in the drawer of my bedside table, I didn't offer the boys anything other than the occasional bottle of Mythos at Café Pushkin, a couple of cartons of cigarettes, and a few phone cards. If I knew what to buy, I'd buy it immediately. Erica has figured that out, and on the morning of her departure she lays it on the line: "Emmanuel, I suppose you're richer than I am . . ." "You suppose correctly," I confirm, and we agree that I'll pay for her every whim that evening, which suits me fine. The ferry departs at 11 p.m., and at seven o'clock we leave to pick up the boys at the Pikpa. Without knowing how long she'll be gone—about which she remains evasive— I assume Erica will need a taxi for her things. She comes down with a duffel bag slung over her shoulder. "Is that all?" That's all. I'm amazed. As someone who never packs too much and makes a point of not checking any bags, I've met my match. I also admire the fact that unlike everyone else these days, she travels with a bag slung over her shoulder rather than a wheeled suitcase. Such suitcases are practical, okay, but they lack romance. In my view they're one of the least sexy accessories in the world, and my esteem for Erica is further enhanced by this soft canvas bag that I can easily squeeze between my legs on the front of the scooter. When we arrive at the Pikpa, Mohamed and another boy called Hussein, who are in a way the second string of our little group, far behind Hamid and Atiq, are each carrying children on their backs, one a little boy, the other a little girl, the youngest offspring of a very large Syrian family I know but don't really know—I mean I know their names but I get them confused. They play at jousting, the boys being the horses and the children their riders, and they're having the time of their lives. The evening is off to a good start. All four of the boys have gotten dressed up, their trousers and T-shirts are impeccable. Even I, who at this moment in my life take a certain pleasure in being dirty, have put on a clean shirt at Erica's behest. As for Erica, she's wearing one of her snug cocktail dresses that suit the place, the season, and the prospect of a boat ride as badly as they do her lumberjack's body. But I like it, because it's Erica who's wearing it, and I like Erica. I really like her, yes, I really, simply, like her, and I'm beginning to realize that I'm sad she's leaving. We call a taxi and she gets in with Hamid, Hussein, and Mohamed, while I say to Atiq that if he likes he can drive my scooter. His face lights up. I could have offered him this joy long ago, but it never occurred to me, even though he's told me several times how much he liked driving the different motorbikes he bought each year in Quetta. On this point, however, there's no point in lamenting: Atiq is still here, I can lend him the scooter as much as he wants and as much as I want; for once we can avoid the bitter taste of being too slow on the uptake. He's a responsive, safe driver. Sitting behind him in Erica's seat, I lean over his shoulder to tell him I drive so slowly that I'm a legend in my family, and that when they were little my sons declared we should have a party on the historic day when I finally passed a car. Atiq laughs, and with the wind blowing in his hair, he leans back and asks my sons' names. It's practically the first question he's asked me since we met. We had to wait until we were on this scooter together, with him in the dominant driver's seat and me in the sub-ordinate position of passenger, for him to take an interest in me. He asks a couple more questions about my family.

Apart from the fact that a speeding scooter on a winding road isn't the best place to start pouring your heart out, I say to myself that I'm not going to bore him with my sob story right now, so I tell him what I think he wants to hear because it's encouraging, because it's what he's longing for and what I hope he'll get: a family, yes, they're well, they're doing very well. I've got a good life, everything's fine, I've got a nice house, a good job, everything's A-okay—and after all, just a few months ago it was true.

Molenbeek

I didn't take any photos during my stay on Leros, but Erica and the boys took pictures that whole evening and sent me a few. Most of them show the first stop on our night on the town, on the terrace of the fanciest—actually the only fancy—hotel on Leros. The waitress, not particularly thrilled by this table of young refugees, takes our orders reluctantly. She says we can have olives and peanuts only if we order wine or beer, not with orange juice or soft drinks. The boys are intimidated at first by her hostility, but as it's clear that Erica and I couldn't care less and show it, and what's more that we'll have the restaurant's entire supply of olives and peanuts brought to us if we want, they cheer up and grow bolder. These photos show their excitement, their pleasure at being together and leaving their worried torpor behind them for a few hours. The relationship between Atiq and Hamid also reminds me of my favorite Visconti film, *Rocco and His Brothers*. The two main characters, two brothers, are played by Renato Salvatori and Alain Delon. Renato Salvatori is a rather rough-hewn actor, with rustic virility. He's good-looking, sure, but no more than that. Delon, in this film and at this age, is perhaps the most handsome actor in the history of cinema: it's supernatural. Yet the whole film tells us that Renato Salvatori is a monster of charisma: all he has to do is appear and women, men, and animals fall in love with him, while Delon, in the shadow of his overbearing older brother, is the shy, melancholic kid whom everyone ignores. Right from the start, I was struck by Hamid's resemblance to Delon as well as by his melancholy, and by Atiq's vitality and charm, although he's not exactly what you'd call good-looking. Throughout this long aperitif on the terrace we discuss their future, but not the same way as at the Pikpa. There, talking about yourself is like handing in a school assignment, here it's part of a normal conversation, not between students and teachers but between human beings. Hamid, who hopes to join his brother in Bavaria, wants to become an accountant. What Hussein and Mohamed want to do I don't remember—in general I don't remember much about them. As for Atiq, he's expected by his uncle who works in a restaurant and who paid the four thousand dollars for his trip. I've known all this for a long time but for the first time it really interests me, not just in the abstract. For the first time I ask specific questions, just like Atiq asked about me and my family for the first time when he was driving the scooter. I want to know more about the uncle who works in a restaurant: who he is, what he looks like, if he has a family, what kind of food his restaurant serves, if he's an employee or his own boss. My curiosity pleases Atiq, it's as if we're really getting to know each other tonight. His uncle has a family, yes, two children, a twelve-year-old boy, Sadiq, and an eight-year-old girl, Zahra. He has a house, not an apartment, a real house with a garden. Atiq will have his own room and a computer, which he needs because he wants to become a computer programmer. As for the restaurant, Atiq doesn't know if his uncle is the boss or not, and I feel like I've brought up a question he's never really asked himself, which suddenly worries him. Because it's not the same thing, and his future won't be the same, if he's going to stay with an uncle who's got his own business and who reigns, dynamic and debonair, over a small world of bustling waiters and loyal customers, or with a poor guy who's paid under the table to wash dishes in a cockroach-infested kitchen. He looks in his phone for the restaurant's menu, which he shows me. The place is called Solo Mio, it's a pizzeria, which makes it less likely that it's run by an Afghan, but who knows? I look at the address without expecting it to ring any bells because I hardly know Brussels. But the name catches my eye: Atiq's uncle's restaurant is in a district called Molenbeek. And Molenbeek, at least at the time I'm discussing, is known even to people who follow the news as sporadically as I do as a jihadist hotbed. Many of the people who've committed terrorist attacks grew up in Molenbeek, or lived in Molenbeek, or hid out in Molenbeek at one point or another. This reputation is terribly unfair to the majority of Molenbeek's inhabitants, who have nothing to do with jihadism, and Atiq's uncle is certainly part of this peaceful majority. But at this point I can't help thinking that in a group of four or five teenagers as endearing and destitute as ours there might be one who, fed up with being rejected and treated like an outcast everywhere he goes, will stop believing that he has a chance of becoming an accountant in Bavaria or a computer programmer in Belgium, and will get radicalized, as they say, and blow himself up, taking with him as many people like us as he can.

At the pier

From the hotel, we take the taxi that we've chartered for the evening to a restaurant, also chic, down by the water. We order a festive meal, with the best and biggest fish. I drink too much, knowing I'll regret it the next day, but who cares. The time comes for us to go to the port and wait for the ferry. It's August 15, the Feast of the Assumption, and big tables have been set up on the quay. There's a small band and lanterns. Many people, tourists and locals mixed, are dancing the sirtaki. Children shoot off firecrackers. It's very merry. As there's no more room on the café terraces, we sit on the steps of the pier, which isn't made of concrete like most piers but is instead covered with black marble slabs that are beautifully veined and polished by time. Atiq takes off his running shoes. After a few steps, he shrieks with joy and motions to us that we should do the same. Hamid, Hussein, and I take off our shoes as well. We, too, are delighted. Several hours after sunset the slabs still retain their warmth, and it feels incredibly good to walk on them barefoot. We laugh, mime our joy, overdo it a bit. Recovering my old tai chi reflexes, I show the boys how to unroll their feet as slowly as possible on the ground and then transfer the weight from one leg to the other, also as slowly as possible, like pouring honey. They get a kick out of the idea of going as slowly as possible, and take to the game. Only Erica and Mohamed don't join in, because Mohamed has lain down next to Erica and put his head on her lap, like a child. She strokes his face, his hair, for a long time, and he takes her hand and kisses and strokes it for a long time too, and it's obvious that it does her a world of good as well, because she hasn't touched anyone or been touched by anyone for so long. They both feel good. Until this evening I haven't sensed any particular closeness between Erica and the shy Mohamed, but clearly he's the one whom she finds the hardest to leave, and who'll find it the hardest when she leaves. The lights of the ferry appear in the distance. Even though it looks like it's a long way off, we know it'll be here soon and that it's time to say goodbye. Erica calls out to the boys, who gather around her and Mohamed, who's still lying with his head on her lap. She undoes her duffel bag and pulls out four packages, done up in wrapping paper with red ribbons. They open them: a white sweater for Mohamed, fur-lined gloves for Atiq, a scarf for Hamid, a ski hat for Hussein—the warm clothes their parents didn't give them and that they'd so sorely missed on their trip. She asks each of them to try his gift on to make sure it fits. She tells them where they can exchange them if the size isn't right or if they don't like the color, and says they should go with me in case the salesperson isn't polite. I wonder two things: What shop on Leros sells fur-lined gloves and ski hats? And what can be left in Erica's bag now that she's taken out all these gifts? She's off to Australia with little more than what the boys took with them on their way to Europe. The ferry docks with its stern against the pier. As always, I admire the precision and speed of the maneuver, carried out not by a battery of computers but by one driver all alone on the bridge, who docks this floating city better than I could park a Fiat 500. The stopover should last an hour, it's over in ten minutes. Erica gets up, so does Mohamed, he has no choice. She kisses us one after the other. You don't kiss someone the same way if you're saying goodbye for ten days or for a year or forever, but Erica hasn't said anything about how long she'll be gone and we feel it would be inappropriate to ask. When my turn comes, before heading for the ramp with her bag over her shoulder, she says: "I sent you your present. It's nice, you'll see."

Martha

Black and white, wide shot: filmed from the wings of a concert hall, the image shows a woman from behind, sitting at a piano in a black dress with white polka dots. She puts her fingers on the keys and starts to play. I've listened to the "Heroic" Polonaise enough lately to recognize it from the first bar. Second shot: fingers running across the keys. In all there are only three angles, the third is of the pianist's face from the front. She's very young and stunningly beautiful—as beautiful as the young Delon in *Rocco and His Brothers*. I recognize her immediately, because she's one of my favorite pianists, and not only of mine. It's Martha Argerich. She must be twenty, maybe younger, and she already has that mane of black hair that she never ties back and that she'll have all her life. Her nose is straight, her lips full, her eyelids low and heavy. She's wild, sensual, intense, untamed, dazzling. I listen to her, watch her, all the time wondering why Erica sent me the link to this video before she left, with no other comment than the subject line: 5:30. The cursor indicates that the video is 6:40 long. I now know the "Heroic" Polonaise by heart, I can run through it in my head from beginning to end. That leaves me free to marvel at Martha Argerich's playing, which is very fast (6:40 is slower than Horowitz, but faster than all the rest) but never hurried, incredibly powerful and ethereal. Watching her fingers run across the keys is a delight, but it's nothing compared with the expressions that run across her face as the music progresses. Extreme concentration, extreme abandon. At 4:30, we reach the little note that's way up in the sky, from which the garland unfurls. I hold my breath as Martha Argerich unfurls it. She's in a kind of languid, suspended trance. Chopin's dynamic marking for this passage is *smorzando*, a very rare indication that means: fading away. Martha Argerich fades away live, letting these dreamlike notes flow, but she knows—and we know—that at this point the grand theme of the polonaise will return and that this radiant return is the high point of the piece. The time reads 5:15, fifteen seconds before 5:30, the time Erica indicated to me in the subject line. I wonder what's going to happen, and here's what happens: we're at the last notes of the garland before the theme returns, grand and joyful, from the right side of the keyboard and the right side of the screen. Carried by this return, Martha Argerich rides it like a surfer on a wave. Abandoning herself to it completely, she can no longer stay in the frame, she jerks her head and leaves the frame to the left with her mass of black hair, disappearing for a moment. And when she comes back into the frame she has a smile on her lips. And at that moment . . . This little girl's smile that comes both from childhood and from the music, this smile of pure joy, lasts exactly five seconds, from 5:30 to 5:35, but during these five seconds we have a glimpse of paradise. She was there, for five seconds, but five seconds are enough, and by watching her we have access to it. Access by proxy, but access nonetheless. We know it exists.

What's on the left

As Erica predicted, I watched this video a lot in the days after she left. I still listen to it and watch it often. I show it to people I love. I assume that after reading the previous chapter, you've typed in "martha argerich heroic polonaise," and that you've watched it as well. Maybe it makes you feel good too. Maybe you also send the link to people you love. As Hervé says, it reminds us that there's an open side to things. Google's algorithm refers people who've watched and liked this video to a documentary on the pianist made by her daughter, who, while admiring her mother no end, has good reasons for resenting her as a neurotic, despotic, toxic mother who's as dreadful as she is powerful. It's rather comforting to know that the heavens are open not only to the saints, the sages, and the zafu devotees, but also to us members of the magnificent and lamentable family of the nervous, those beset by the black dogs. Every time I see Martha Argerich leaving the frame to the left, just before the grand and joyful theme of the polonaise returns, as if she were going to look for something far behind her in the darkness, and then coming back with this smile of pure joy, of course I think of Erica and what these images mean to her. It's the story of her life: going to look for the shadow on her left, the shadow and the madness and the disappearance of Claire, who's vanished somewhere to her left, who continues to live somewhere to her left, at the limit of her field of vision, so close and forever out of reach. And taken together, what this music and Martha Argerich's twenty-year-old face say to her, and what she's saying to me in turn, is that from this left side where Claire has disappeared you can return alive, fully alive. There's the shadow, but there's also pure joy, and perhaps there can be no pure joy without a shadow, and in that case it's worth living with the shadow. Erica's gift is to tell me that pure joy is as real as the shadow. Not more real, no, but just as real, and that's already a lot. And for someone like me who believes that ultimate reality, the bottom line, is Raoul Dufy's abominable little seascape, that's good news.

A stagnant estuary of my life

Erica had said I could use her room while she was away, so I went upstairs with my bag. I've seen this room only once, when she showed me around the place on my arrival. It seemed nice, and it is: spacious, open on three sides, with a small terrace and a view. But I stayed in my children's room. I kept sleeping in my tiny single bed. I went from sleeping not much and badly to sleeping badly but a lot. My days were all the same: waking up late, a cup of tea and then a bit of yoga on the terrace, coffee in the port, after which I went to the Pikpa. With Erica gone, the workshop had lost all introspective and therapeutic ambition and become an English class with essays on harmless topics, but I took it seriously. Then I'd go down to the beach, float on my back in the water, and have a nap. I'd lie on the sand until dinner, which I invariably had at Café Pushkin, chatting with Svetlana Sergeyevna, who'd become my main contact. She's not Russian, in fact, but Belarusian, from Pripyat, the little town that the world first heard of in 1986 because it was closest to the Chernobyl nuclear power plant. A cousin of Svetlana's was one of the technicians who built the sarcophagus to cover the reactor, and he died a few months later in a horrific manner, his whole body falling apart. Many of her family members developed cancer, and a neighbor gave birth to a baby boy who looked like a bag with no eyes or ears, a slit for a mouth, and no anus. During the first months of his life, she wondered what words she would find when the time came to explain to him why he was like that, why he would never know love, why God had allowed such misfortune. Luckily he died very quickly. How kind God has been to me! I thought of my own children, so beautiful, so gifted, so alive. Except for a few messages to Jeanne, I didn't give anyone any news and didn't expect any either. I didn't send or receive emails, I didn't listen to my messages. And I didn't hear from Erica. I was doing badly, but better than before. I felt far from everything, as if I'd fallen into a stagnant estuary of my life, and in a strange way, I felt safe. I flirted a bit in vain with one of the pretty Italian twins who worked as volunteers at the Pikpa. In her real life she studied at the Scuola Holden, a school of narrative techniques founded by the Italian writer Alessandro Baricco, the crème de la crème of creative writing schools. I asked Susanna—her name is Susanna—why, if writing was her vocation, she wasn't teaching it here, instead of gardening. She said she didn't feel ready for it, and I said that in that case she never would be: that made her think. I rented a

second scooter for Atiq and we took a few spins around
the island together. I wanted to take the boys to the beach,
which after all is the best thing you can do on a Greek
island, but they kept hemming and hawing and coming up
with reasons not to go. The real reason, I think, is that they
don't know how to swim.

Seen from the sky

One evening I had dinner with Elfriede and Moritz, the
Austrian archaeologist couple, and I felt bad about casting
Moritz as a sadistic Haneke character because I'm ready to
swear that he's open-minded, young at heart, and doesn't
have a mean bone in his body. And the same goes for Elfriede. This dinner at Café Pushkin was not only friendly
but also very instructive, as during their stay Elfriede and
Moritz had become interested in the island's past and in
particular its architecture, which is so foreign to the style of
the Greek islands, and which I'd been intrigued by on my
arrival without trying to find out more. During the Italian
occupation in the thirties, Elfriede and Moritz explained to
me, speaking in turn, one starting a sentence and the other
finishing it with touching unison, there was a plan to make
Leros a naval base. Mussolini sent in two eminent repre-
sentatives of Fascist architecture who built large, modernist
buildings like the Pikpa, as well as a hundred or so pavilions arranged in concentric circles to house the garrison.
After the war this utopian-style city remained deserted until the sixties, when it became first a detention and torture

center for political prisoners under the junta known as the Regime of the Colonels, and then, when the colonels were overthrown, a psychiatric hospital, the largest in the country, holding as many patients as the base would have held sailors and their families, so a good thousand people or so. Everyone knew that the patients in this hospital were treated abominably. Naked most of the time and left to soak in their own piss and shit, they were washed once a week with a hose in the courtyard and abused by the orderlies—all islanders, for whom the hospital was the major and practically the only employer. After thirty years of operation and following a report in which the philosopher and psychiatrist Félix Guattari called the institution the shame of European psychiatry, the wards were closed, the nutcases dispersed, and the abandoned utopian city took on that deserted, silent look, crushed by a sun without warmth, that reminded me of the paintings of Giorgio de Chirico. Then the refugee crisis revived it. The migrants were stationed where the nutcases once were, and the islanders who used to work as orderlies began to work for the NGOs, which in turn became the main employers on Leros. Elfriede and Moritz's story gave me food for thought, because the four layers of the island's history they described went a long way toward explaining the strange vibes I'd been getting since I arrived. When I said that, they both laughed, because that wasn't all, they went on. At the end of the war there was also a very brief German occupation, a fifth layer of history lasting only a few months, and of which only one vestige remained: a sort of bas-relief about ten meters in diameter, engraved in a rocky outcrop at the very tip of the island, visible only from the air. But if you fly over Leros in a helicopter it's the first thing you see, and that thing is a swastika.

The longest-residing guest

As the summer drew to a close, Elfriede and Moritz returned to Vienna, like Erica not without giving modest but remarkably imaginative gifts, a different, personalized little something for each recipient. Susanna and Roberta, the pretty twins, also left. I was tempted to ask Susanna to give my regards to Baricco, whom I know a little, but didn't in the end. And all things considered I feel it's to my credit that I refrained from such name-dropping in my fruitless attempt at seduction. After this wave of departures, I began to imagine myself becoming a sort of permanent fixture at the Pikpa, like the ghostly figure that another writer I love, Geoff Dyer, describes so well: the longest-residing guest. He writes:

> I was the only person conscious of this status, for the simple reason that no one else had been there as long. If you arrived on a Tuesday, say, you simply saw that a number of guests had already settled in by the time you arrived. You could not have known that I had seen them all arrive, even as you had now arrived, and would see them depart, even as I would see you depart . . .

I didn't expect anything more from my stay, but I didn't see any particular reason to end it either. One day, however, something happened. It was lunchtime. As always, the aluminum foil containers filled with rice had been distributed, served that day with fish. I was eating alone in the shade of the big plane tree, watching absentmindedly as Hamid played with three kids from the large Syrian family at the back of the courtyard. Hamid is always very kind to them, he's truly interested in the things that interest them, and they adore him of course. I watched as they shifted their weight very slowly from one leg to the other under his guidance, laughing at their own slowness, and I realized that Hamid was teaching them tai chi. All he knew was the few movements I'd taught him in not even five minutes on the warm, smooth marble of the pier the night Erica left. Nevertheless, with no more than that you can practice for a good while. Hamid and his little students were clearly delighted, and I thought there might be something we could try.

Hamid teaches

Although I didn't formally open a tai chi workshop and list it in the schedule, a small group of us got together to practice in the courtyard every day. The mainstays were Atiq and Hamid, Mohamed sometimes, and the Syrian children. I was a bit surprised because the idea seems a little abstract, but they all loved the game of finding the longest distance between two points. They started going round and round in long loops, sometimes with their eyes closed. The problem was to measure the distance each one covered, but for that there are apps that everyone with a smartphone downloaded. It was fun to watch the children walking around the playground in slow motion, both very serious and close to breaking into fits of laughter at any moment. I thought back to the walks on the fenced path of the Vipassana center in the Morvan region, and it struck me that what we were improvising here at the Pikpa in a playful, ad hoc way was closer to real meditation than sitting on our zafus and focusing endlessly on the insides of our nostrils. But as soon as I thought that, I also thought: who knows, maybe focusing on our nostrils could catch on here as well. And I wasn't wrong. It'd be an exaggeration to say that everyone at the Pikpa immediately took to observing the flow of air in their nostrils, but the exercise intrigued Hamid, it intrigued Mohamed, and it intrigued Elias and Dina, two of the Syrian children. It intrigued them and above all it made them laugh. For them it was a new twist to the game all children love to play: blocking your nose and holding your breath for as long as you can. All of this worked so well, I think, because it was no longer me teaching but Hamid, whom the children idolized, as I've said. Each time we drank a Mythos at Café Pushkin I'd casually run over a thing or two. Then we'd go down to the dock where Svetlana Sergeyevna's customers moor their boats and I'd show him a move that we'd practice together, as I'd practiced with the Canadian Father Christmas to tame the wolf, after which I'd sit at the foot of the big plane tree and watch Hamid, listening to him from a distance: "As if you pour honey inside your leg . . ." He was a wonderful teacher.

Thirty years for nothing?

Apart from George Langelaan's short story I hadn't read anything for months, but one day in Café Pushkin I opened the cardboard folder on which I'd written *Exhaling* in capital letters, and started—not really to read—let's say to skim through the fifty thousand or so words of notes on yoga, tai chi, and meditation: the pastimes that have occupied me for half of my life, and all for what? The answer was enough to bring me down. Thirty years of pursuing calm and strategic depth, thirty years of seeing my life as a way out of confusion and as the patient construction of a state of wonder and serenity, thirty years of believing in all of this despite numerous setbacks and depressions, and at the end of the day, as I approached old age, although I had a home, a family, everything you need to be wise and happy, I found myself lying curled up in a tiny bed, alone in the empty house of a lonely, lost woman who had left without leaving an address, she too for somewhere in the Southern Hemisphere. It wasn't a great track record. And it's not very good publicity for yoga. But that's not entirely true: the problem isn't with yoga, it's with me. Yoga aims to achieve unity, I'm too divided for that. One day while walking on the mountain paths above Le Levron, Hervé and I asked ourselves: Can everyone do yoga? Does everyone have access to the unity, the light, the secret, radiant zone inside themselves? At the time we concluded that yes, this access may be hidden but it exists for everyone, otherwise yoga wouldn't be yoga. That way of thinking strives toward a happy ending. But you have to wonder: Can a schizophrenic like Erica's sister do yoga? Someone who's shattered to the core? Someone like me, one half of whom is enemy to the other?

The good old dogs

These thoughts are melancholic, but they weren't painful. They didn't prevent me from going about my daily routine, helping Hamid prepare the tai chi lessons he gave to the Syrian children, or leading a life without projects, which was restful for precisely that reason. I felt like a wounded soldier who's not unhappy to find himself tucked away in a ramshackle, poorly run but halfway cushy hospital. Sitting in my rattan armchair in Café Pushkin and sipping my Mythos beer, I let my poor, frayed thoughts peacefully permeate my mind. I watched them flow past without paying too much attention. The most haunting, toxic ones I knew by heart, and when I saw them coming they no longer seemed like demons trying to devour my soul, but like good old dogs that are a bit clumsy and a bit of a nuisance—like the mongrel we called "the poor old guy" whom my boys loved so much during our summers at Pointe de l'Arcouest— and who are forever pawing you and licking you and trying to get you to throw them a stick, which they bring back panting, wagging their tails and wanting to start all over again. So I'd throw them their sticks again and again, the stick of vanity, the stick of self-hatred, the stick of being too slow on the uptake and of the bitter taste that leaves behind. And then at one point I'd say that's enough, and retreat once more into my drowsy state, leaving the good

old annoying dogs circling around me, a bit disappointed.
After starting to sleep a lot, I also started to sleep well. I
slept in my bed, I slept at the beach, I slept at the café.
The good old dogs growled while half asleep. Napping had
become our form of meditation.

Pissing and shitting

This form of meditation is missing from the list of definitions I've accumulated in my yoga file. I was too lazy to study
these pages seriously, but I thought that a good way to skim
through them would be to list the definitions, which are as
follows: Meditation is sitting silent and motionless. Meditation is everything that happens in your consciousness while
you're sitting silent and motionless. Meditation is creating a
witness inside you who monitors the whirlwind of thoughts
without being swept away by them. Meditation is seeing
things as they are. Meditation is detaching from what you
call yourself. Meditation is discovering that you're something other than the thing that is relentlessly saying: Me!
Me! Me! Meditation is discovering that you are something
other than your ego. Meditation is a technique for dimin-
ishing your ego. Meditation is diving and settling into what
is bothersome in life. Meditation is not judging. Meditation is paying attention. Meditation is observing the points
of contact between what is oneself and what is not oneself.
Meditation is stopping the fluctuations of the mind. Meditation is observing these fluctuations called vritti, calming
them, and eventually making them disappear. Meditation is

being aware that others exist. Meditation is diving within yourself and digging tunnels, building dams, opening lanes, bringing something into being and out into the open sky. Meditation is finding a secret, radiant zone within you, where you feel good. Meditation is being in your place, wherever you are. Meditation is being aware of everything, all the time (this is Krishnamurti's definition). Meditation is accepting what comes. Meditation is not telling yourself stories. Meditation is letting go, not expecting anything, not trying to do anything. Meditation is living in the present moment. Meditation is pissing and shitting when you piss and shit, nothing more. Meditation is not adding anything. That's it. I've read and reread this list of definitions, and I can let them stand like that. Apart from Krishnamurti's, they don't come from books but from firsthand experience on my own small level. Is there one that encompasses all the others? One that's more general than the rest? One that would look like the mountain when you've reached the end of the journey? Do you remember? At the beginning of the journey, the distant mountain looks like a mountain. As the journey unfolds, it looks like a thousand things but no longer like a mountain. And at the end of the journey, it looks like a mountain once again, but differently: it *really is* the mountain. How far have I come on the journey? Am I close to the mountain, or am I still a long way off? And if I had to choose just one of these definitions, which would it be? It depends on the moment. Today, in the early autumn of 2016, as I put off my departure from Leros with no more reason to leave than to stay, I tend to prefer: meditation is pissing when you piss and shitting when you shit. As that pretty well sums up what I'm doing here, without going into too much detail, I sometimes get the amused impression that I'm really, finally, meditating. I'm neither happy nor sad, I throw the good old dogs their sticks, the stick of vanity, the stick of self-hatred, the stick of being too slow on the uptake and of the bitter taste that leaves behind, and it's quite surprising, but the fact is that I almost feel good.

V

I CONTINUE NOT TO DIE

Paul in Guadalajara

The last time I saw Paul Otchakovsky-Laurens, who'd been my publisher for the past thirty-five years, was in November 2017 at the Guadalajara Book Fair in Mexico, where we were both invited guests. He came with his wife, Emmie Landon, who's also one of my best friends, and has been for almost as long. A little more than a year after my return from Leros I was feeling much better, and the three of us had a great time. A short video shows us in a cantina with other friends, writers and publishers from all over, laughing, talking nonsense, and letting off steam like all conventioneers do once their conferences and round tables are over. It shows Paul and Emmie looking at each other the way they used to look at each other, and the way I've never seen any other couple look at each other in my life— I know, I said the same thing about Bernard and Hélène, but Bernard and Hélène had just met, whereas for Paul and

Emmie the enchantment of the early days of love had lasted
unbroken for twenty years. It also shows Paul turned toward me and talking as if he was trying to convince me of
something, which is exactly what he was doing, because it
was just before we joined this merry group that the little
scene that is the subject of this chapter took place. Paul,
Emmie, and I had arranged to meet at the hotel bar. I go
down first, take my tablet from my pack, and take advantage of what one of my friends calls "interstitial time" (she
hates such unattributed moments, I like them) to answer
some emails. Paul joins me and I tell him I'll just be a sec.
"Take your time," he says, "there's no rush," and he starts
tapping away on his phone. A little interstitial time goes by,
suddenly interrupted by Paul's stunned, almost shocked
voice: "Emmanuel, what are you *doing*? How are you typing?" I look up, not really following. "Tell me it's not true:
Are you typing *with one finger*?" "Yes, I'm typing with one
finger. I've always typed with one finger." "Now, wait a minute," Paul goes on with growing amazement, as if he was
gradually becoming aware of just how outrageous this was,
"do you mean to say that you've written all of your books,
not to mention all your articles and screenplays, *with just
one finger*?" Later, after Paul's death, Emmie told me that
he typed very well, without looking at the keyboard or the
screen, and that he was proud of this skill—a skill I had
ignored, just as he had ignored my lack of skill until that
night in Guadalajara. But he discovered it that night, and
this revelation plunges him into a sort of giddy amazement
that must be similar, I think, to what you feel after eating
magic mushrooms. We've known each other for thirty-five

years, he's published twelve of my books, he's the godfather of my son Gabriel, who for that reason will receive all the books published by P.O.L for the rest of his life, we've gone on vacation together, and what he never knew was that I type with just one finger, my right index finger, without even using my left index finger or my thumb for the space bar. After the first wave of hallucinogenic laughter and bewilderment, it's time for questions and attempts at an explanation. Paul can't understand why I haven't learned to type, and I say that now that I think about it, yes, I admit it is a bit surprising. Really. Sure, I could have learned. But what's no less sure is that I didn't. That's just how it is. Until tonight no one's been particularly alarmed by the fact. None of the women I've lived with have shown this kind of astonishment. I'm not saying they didn't notice, of course they did, but for them, as for my children, the fact that I type with one finger has always been the stuff of affectionate jokes, like the fact that I drive very slowly and that even on the highway I shift into fourth gear about as often as I use the ejector seat. It's the subject of loving jibes I'm happy to go along with, but no more than that. No one's told me that I could learn, or that I should learn, or that above all, seeing as it was my job to type, it could be useful and even life-changing if I learned to do it properly. Why didn't I learn? It certainly wasn't a principled hostility to innovation or technology, even if I'm not about to go out and break a lance for either one. I don't know how to explain it, but it's just that as far as typing goes, it never happened. The opportunity never presented itself, and then I learned to get by without it. A bit like people who don't get their driver's license when they reach driving age and then the moment goes by, it's too late. "Sure," Paul objects to my objection, "except that with you it's like (a) you don't know how to drive, and (b) you're a Formula One champion." In the hours that followed he shared his discovery with Emmie, who was no less amused by it, and then with anyone who'd listen over dinner. He didn't let up with me either, and at one point the precious little video that's the last image I have of him shows him leaning toward me, looking like he was fervently hammering in a point, and in fact I remember just how fervently he insisted all evening that I should learn to type. He even took out his phone to look for a method—"This looks perfect: typing.com!"—and I said yes, maybe, why not, but at the same time, what's the point? I've reached the age of sixty, everything I've written I've written with one finger, it's too late to change now, and besides, what would it change if I changed? Paul was undeterred: "You don't realize how much time it'll save you." This argument about saving time was a nonstarter: you don't write books to save time. And Paul, who knew this better than anyone, quickly abandoned that tack. We dropped the subject, for a while he seemed resigned to me persisting in my incompetence, and it was only later in the evening when we went to a second, darker, busier, noisier cantina and switched from tequila to mezcal that at one point, as we were leaning against the bar, Paul turned to me, his eyes shining—I'll have to write about the way Paul's eyes shone—and said, shouting over the noise: "You know, if you learned to type, you wouldn't just write faster, you'd write *differently*."

"The most important act in your life"

Like me, Paul was a sentimental and effusive drinker, very Russian. And like me, he sometimes wondered the next morning if he hadn't gone too far the night before, resulting in convoluted, overly delicate phone calls. We didn't need to phone each other in Guadalajara because we saw each other from morning to night for the whole four days, but the next day at lunch—one of those more or less official dos where you try to get around the seating plan and sit with your friends—he asked me with that worried, post-booze-up look I knew so well if I hadn't taken what he'd said to me in the cantina the wrong way, and if I hadn't concluded that in his view my books could be ten times better, meaning that logically they were ten times worse than they could have been if I'd gone to the trouble of learning how to type. I told Paul that I hadn't taken it badly at all, but the fact was that he had said exactly that, we both had, leaning against the bar of the cantina after switching from tequila to mezcal—because I was still drinking back then, and it suddenly occurs to me that without having ever decided or made the connection, it was after Paul's death that I stopped drinking entirely, and I think for good. From the moment we went from "you'd write faster" to "you'd write *differently*," a gamut of alcoholic speculation opened up. "Typing on a keyboard," Paul argued at the bar, "transforming your thoughts into words and sentences that you type on a keyboard, is the most important act in your life. If you change the conditions of this act, it cannot remain without consequences. It will inevitably change something in your way of writing, it'll create new neural connections. Yes, you'll write differently, you cannot not write differently." It was at this moment of drunkenness that it struck us like a bolt from the blue that what I would write with ten fingers would be ten times better than what I wrote with just one. I'd brushed off the speed argument, saying that I didn't care about typing fast, but in fact I do, because I belong to the species of writers who are mainly occupied with transcribing what comes into their heads—a task that requires both patience and speed. It's not very complicated to write, Thomas Bernhard has been quoted as saying, all you have to do is tilt your head and drop everything onto a sheet of paper. Okay, but to catch as much as possible of what comes out it's good to go fast, and after a moment of skepticism I enthusiastically welcomed the idea, typical of Paul, that there was a technical solution, one open to us precisely because it was technical, that allowed us to progress in this art. I say "typical of Paul," and I add typical of me, too, because the two of us shared not only a taste for drunken outpourings but also the conviction that people are on earth to improve themselves, and that it's possible to improve yourself whatever your "available material," as Lenin said, as long as you go about it seriously and assiduously. This trait, when you think about it, isn't as widespread as all that, it's another one of the borders that divides humanity into two classes. Almost everyone has an ideal self, a better version of themselves, but only a particular category of people tries to approach this ideal and make it less ephemeral by practicing what Montaigne and the ancients before him called exercise—or *meditatio*.

Paul practiced neither meditation nor yoga, but he did do two hundred push-ups every day at dawn. All his life he got up at daybreak, and even before daybreak. This monotonous way of exercising was the source of affectionate jokes for our friend Olivier Rubinstein and me: push-ups and only push-ups, like a one-food diet, which gave him an extremely powerful torso on spindly legs—but it was clear that Emmie was fine with the result and nothing else mattered to Paul. And although he practiced neither meditation nor yoga, when I told him about my yoga book project, instead of shrugging his shoulders in mildly ironic bafflement as most of my friends have done the whole time I've been working on this book, he showed true unjaded curiosity—not just, I think, because he was interested in my projects as a matter of principle but because he was generally interested in all disciplines aimed at forming the soul. And it's for that reason that I find it both surprising and not surprising that before he died, he left me as a last gift the conviction that typing correctly, with my ten fingers, could be my personal and ultimate form of yoga.

The way his eyes shone

Paul died on January 2, 2018, on a small road in Guadeloupe where he was on vacation with Emmie. He was seventy-three years old, with the silhouette and all the enthusiasm of a teenager, and he was madly in love. I think, and I've always thought, that for each of us there are a few people, it could be five, it could be ten, not many more, with whom we go through life. Together with Emmie, Hervé, Olivier, Ruth, and François, Paul was one of those people for me, part of the small, essential group of those with whom we make the crossing, and his death was the first great loss of my life, which had been surprisingly preserved in this respect. The first novel I wrote I sent to him, and to him alone, without knowing him, because P.O.L published Georges Perec. Since 1984 he's put out all my books, and it's very strange for me to finish this one knowing that he won't be reading it. I'm sometimes asked how we worked together, what kind of comments he made on my manuscripts, whether he changed much . . . Actually, not so much. Paul saw a book as something organic, to be taken or left, and not to be put through an editing mill. He was convinced that what we take to be flaws when they're under our noses often turn out with hindsight to be what makes a book unique and inimitable. So of course he made comments, and good ones, but other people can, and do, and will make good comments: it wasn't his good comments that made Paul unique for me. What made Paul unique for me was the way his eyes shone when I brought him a manuscript. It was a certainty that he would read it *immediately* and call me in the middle of the night when he'd finished it, and that if he didn't call me in the middle of the night it would mean that he was dead—and that's how it is now. Paul won't call me in the middle of the night because he's dead. I will have, I do have another editor, Frédéric Boyer, whom I've known for twenty years. Like me, he's an author at P.O.L, and he's a friend, but never again will anyone *desire* what I write the way Paul desired it. And I'm not the only one who can say that. Of course, our relationship was special: we'd made our lives together, we were close friends, we knew if not everything, at least a lot about each other. But I think all the authors he published knew the way his eyes shone—otherwise he wouldn't have published them. That, too, was one of the things that made this small publishing house and its founder so extraordinary: authors whose books sold five hundred copies throughout their careers were accorded the same respect and exacting loyalty as those whose larger print runs kept the shop going. Paul's eyes shone for their books just as lovingly. And just as jealously, just as possessively, too, because Paul was also jealous and possessive. And it would be a pity at this point, I feel, to pass over in silence the enchanting story of *An Elegy for Chamalières* and its author, Renaud Camus. Please don't be angry. Don't put on your coat and leave, slamming the door behind you. Sit back down. If you know who he is, you will think the worst of Renaud Camus, and so do I, I swear, don't worry. If you don't know who he is, let's say straight off that he's now a far-right ideologist, inventor of the theory of the "great replacement" (of good old French people by Blacks and Arabs) and an inspiration for white supremacists who, from New Zealand to Norway, perpetrate shootings at mosques in the name of his doctrine. That said, it's interesting to know that up until the end of the last century, Renaud Camus was a writer for the avant-garde happy few. He rubbed shoulders with the likes of Roland Barthes and Andy Warhol, was known for a timeless gay-lit classic, *Tricks*, and for a monumental *Diary*, which Paul published unfailingly year after year—and of which I was

an unfailing reader. I'll put my head on the block and say
that Renaud Camus was an exceptional writer, and that
his current folly can't change that, what's done is done. We
were friends at the time, and we were two pillars of Édi-
tions P.O.L, you could even say we were part of its DNA.
Here's what happened. Until he broke with him in 1999,
Paul published *everything* Renaud Camus wrote, at least
fifty volumes, which delighted a very small circle of readers
without bringing in a cent, and which even cost money to
publish, but Paul didn't care, as far as he was concerned
Renaud Camus was a great writer and his job was to publish a great writer when he saw one, and what's more to
publish *everything* that great writer wrote. Now, one day
Renaud Camus, who lives in a run-down château deep in
southwestern France, accepts the proposal of a small publisher who specializes in local erudition, and what's more
is his neighbor, to write a booklet of about thirty pages
entitled *An Elegy for Chamalières*, because like the former
president Giscard d'Estaing, Renaud Camus is a native of
the town of Chamalières in the Auvergne region. As a publication it's so modest, so discreet, so local in nature that in
all good faith Renaud Camus doesn't even think of letting
Paul, his main publisher, know. But Paul finds out and it
drives him mad. He summons Renaud Camus to Paris, because the two of them have to talk. "You know what's terrible about this, Renaud?" he says to Renaud Camus without
giving him time to sit down. "The terrible thing, the thing
that really makes me sick, is not only that you published
An Elegy for Chamalières with another house. It's that *An
Elegy for Chamalières*, and you know this very well, is your

most beautiful book." Renaud wasn't expecting that, he himself would never have thought that this booklet, jotted down in a single afternoon, and which he took on more to get in good with a neighbor than to make any special contribution to literature, could be ranked so high in his oeuvre. But it would be underestimating Paul to imagine that he'd stop there. "You've read—or seen—*Fahrenheit 451*, right? Do you remember the story? The world where books are banned, where the state burns books? Do you remember that in this world there are groups of resistance fighters who hide out and learn the forbidden books by heart? Each one learns one, and only one, and is named after it. He's no longer called Peter or Paul: no, for eternity his name will be *Gulliver's Travels*, or Ecclesiastes, or *The Life of Samuel Johnson*. Do you remember, Renaud?" Renaud nods, not daring to imagine what'll come next. "Well, you see, Renaud," Paul concludes, "in that world, in the world of *Fahrenheit 451*, my name would be *An Elegy for Chamalières*!" (Now I think you see what I mean when I talk of the way Paul's eyes shone.)

With my ten fingers

I can be reproached for many things, but not for lack of zeal. I'm on vacation on Belle Île, in Brittany, and every day I spend five or six hours shut away in my hotel room, working my way through typing.com, the lessons that Paul recommended to me so fervently in Guadalajara a year and a half ago. I've made it through the first level, the one that shows you where the letters are placed without yet going as far as forming words. I've got my head around the first eight keys, the ones in the middle line: a, s, d, f on the left, and j, k, l, ; on the right, with the little ridges at the bottom of the f and j keys. I've added the two middle letters, g and h, which I reach with the left and right index fingers, the former from its base camp on the f key, the latter from its base camp on the j. That took a lot of time and a huge amount of effort, I went through terrible moments of discouragement at the idea that two more lines of letters awaited me, and then the number keys, then the capitals, not to mention the more remote keys like] and \, as well as things I've never used in my life and about which I know about as much, say, as I do about neutrons and protons: "keyboard short-cuts." Nevertheless I continued, encouraged by comments like "awesome typing!" and little avatars who congratulated me on being a "keyboard warrior" and a "fiery typist" as the lessons progressed. Along the way my left pinkie has learned to reach up to the q above the a and down to the z below it, and up beyond q to the ~ and ! (I often confuse the two), and finally to the Tab, Caps Lock, left Shift, and left Ctrl keys. As for my right pinkie, it controls, among others, the -, =, p, [, ;, ', and / keys. Good use of your pin-kies is the sign that you've joined the closed circle of typ-ists who really use their ten fingers. It's a revolution, and a prelude to two more revolutions: typing without looking at the keyboard and typing without looking at the screen—as Paul could do and as I will probably never be able to do. I have not reached and no doubt will never reach these heights, but I'm progressing, the way you always progress when you work. That's how it is with all learning: the form of tai chi, yoga postures, and of course the piano, which I suppose is similar as it also involves mastering a keyboard. Things that seemed impossible, completely and definitively out of reach, become possible little by little, almost without your noticing it. With my ten clumsy fingers, I've gradually moved from letters to words, then from words to sentences, from sentences to paragraphs, and now from paragraphs to the text. In other words—although I dare say it only when her back is turned—to literature.

"I'm not writing, my friends: I'm doing typing exercises"

If I took a hotel room on Belle Île it's because Ruth and Olivier have rented a house here, and by being close to them I have both the pleasure of solitude and the pleasure of their company. When I join them on the beach or—almost every evening—invite myself to dinner at their place, they ask me if I'm doing well, if I'm happy, and I can see that they're happy, because after more than three years of depression and drifting that they witnessed firsthand, it seems that I'm not only better, but that I've started writing again. What else could a writer be doing for six hours a day, shut up in his room while everyone else is swimming or going for a stroll? Playing patience? Video games? Nevertheless I hold to my story and exclaim: "You're way off the mark! If I shut myself away for six hours a day with my computer it's not to write a book—I'm not ready for that, believe me—it's just to type. Don't be fooled. I'm not writing, my friends: I'm doing typing exercises."

"All work and no play makes Jack a dull boy"

"What sort of typing exercises are you doing?" Olivier asks with a wry smile. "All work and no play makes Jack a dull boy?" Remember that? In *The Shining*, the terrifying mantra of Jack Torrance, the failed writer who accepts a job as off-season caretaker of the huge Overlook Hotel. Cut off from everything during the winter, he settles in with his wife and little boy, hoping that the isolation and forced leisure will allow him to finish the work he's been half-heartedly dragging around with him for years. Every morning he retires to one of the hotel lounges and, like me in my room on Belle Île, spends several hours typing. His wife asks him if he's doing well, if he's happy, and he answers that he is, but he doesn't seem to be doing well at all, he doesn't seem happy at all. His face is increasingly menacing, Jack Nicholson's gabled eyebrows arch more and more devilishly, and his repeated visits to the dreadful room 237 are clearly not helping his mental balance. His wife becomes so worried that she slips into his huge office in his absence and looks at the sheet of paper in the carriage of his typewriter. On it, this one sentence: "All work and no play makes Jack a dull boy." This sentence chills the blood because of what it says, because of its threatening, nursery-rhyme rhythm, and because it's repeated twenty or thirty times on the sheet of paper in the typewriter, but also hundreds, thousands of times on the sheets of paper in a pile beside it. Hundreds, perhaps thousands of sheets of paper covered by this sentence repeated ad infinitum: "All work and no play makes Jack a dull boy."

The assembly cut

The terrifying mantra of *The Shining* has stayed with me all my life. More than once I've identified with the film's pathetic hero. I've known his overbearing dryness, his terror, his cruelty, his grim, self-engulfing madness. Looking in the mirror, I've seen myself pulling the same faces as him. But not this summer. This summer I blithely accept Olivier's jibe. Because protected by my new mantra—you remember: *I'm not writing, I'm doing typing exercises*—I've started to recopy and put together the seemingly disparate files that will make up the book you're reading: one on Vipassana and yoga, one on the days surrounding the *Charlie Hebdo* attack, one on my depression and hospitalization at Sainte-Anne, one on my stay on Leros. Arranging things end to end like this is the first step when you edit a film. In cinema jargon this first version is called the assembly cut, and nobody in their right mind can believe it'll result in something watchable—or readable if it's a book. And then, once you've overcome the urge to toss the whole thing out, you get down to work, you assemble, juxtapose, cut, add, swap, and try things out . . . Little by little this magma starts to resemble something, often something you hadn't planned. Some artists like it when it doesn't correspond to what they'd planned, others don't, it makes them unhappy. There are two families. François Truffaut said that a film is a process of loss. The gap between the idea you had before starting it and the final result can be bigger or smaller: if it's small, the film is successful, if it's big, it's botched. That's what the artists of control think, the demiurges like Hitchcock and Kubrick who want to bend reality to match their will and dreams. For others—including myself—the opposite is the case: the less the film or book resembles what they'd imagined, the longer and more unpredictable the path between the starting point and the end, the more the result surprises them, the happier they are. It's the journey that counts, not where it takes you—or, as Chögyam Trungpa said: "The path is the goal." A lot of unpredictable things have happened, some of them terrible, between my initial project of an upbeat, subtle little book on yoga and what I started to piece together in my hotel room on Belle Île under the pretext of doing typing exercises. And now six months have passed, the book is finished. Well, almost finished. I still have to give it a sort of epilogue, close a few parentheses that I can't reasonably leave open, and sweep up before closing shop. Time to tidy up, put some things away, get rid of others, and close up. Let's start with Leros.

Sitting for a minute in silence

One autumn morning I woke up wanting to leave, something that hadn't even crossed my mind the day before. I returned my scooter, paid a couple of months' rent in advance for Atiq's, said goodbye to everyone at the Pikpa, then locked up the house, left the key in the wooden box containing the electricity meter as Erica had instructed, and took the evening ferry to Athens. On board I realized that I'd left the Samsung Galaxy in the drawer of my bedside table, and wondered who'd open the drawer and when. I never heard from Erica again. She never answered my emails, never posted anything on Facebook. She disappeared, somewhere to the left of the world . . . *She disappeared, somewhere to the left of the world*: that's the kind of cheesy thing you might want to write about a fictional character, the kind of sentence I'd normally cut on the first reading, but on reflection I'd rather keep it, ease my conscience, and admit that Frederica *is* a fictional character. I mean, a partly fictional character. She's modeled on a real person with whom I gave a few lessons at the Pikpa, had a memorable booze-up, and listened to Chopin's "Heroic" Polonaise, but most of the rest is invented. That's what happens, inevitably, I think, as soon as you start changing proper names: fiction takes over and, as my school friend Emmanuel Guilhen used to say, it's the door that opens onto all the windows. It's a question I've often asked myself, in particular when I was writing *The Kingdom*, which deals in part with how the Gospels were written and how Jesus is depicted: Is there a criterion that lets us see whether a story we read is truth or fiction? Whether a painting in a museum depicts a real person or an imaginary one? I don't have an answer, but it seems to me that intuitively, without being able to explain it, we feel it. I can feel it, in any case. Hamid and Atiq have kept their real names, and I follow them on Instagram. One's in Germany, the other in Belgium, they seem to be doing well. They're smiling students, with friends, sports activities, birthday parties, projects. After being quasi-pariahs, they've once again reached the place in society they had back home, and will no doubt become what they wanted to be: accountants and computer programmers. Their perilous journey to Europe and their stay in Leros must be gradually fading from memory, like images from a dream in which I sometimes wonder if there's a place for me. Probably not. If anyone in Leros still thinks of me, I think it's Svetlana Sergeyevna. On the day I left, the two of us sat in Café Pushkin, which was rather dark and deserted at the time. When someone leaves on a trip

in Russia, it's a custom to sit with them for a while and remain silent, each one praying that it won't be the last time,
that God will allow them to see each other again. Then
they get up, kiss each other, and say a quick goodbye. Svetlana Sergeyevna made a sign of the cross on my forehead. I
felt like she was my mother, although she must be slightly
younger than me. I'd like to use this ritual to say goodbye
to this book and wish it—and me, and you, reader—good
luck. Before we turn the last page, which isn't far off, we
could sit together for a minute, close our eyes, and be still.
Don't forget to turn off the light on your way out.

A little salt

Lithium is an alkali metal, an element in the periodic table, and, when administered in salt form, has proved surprisingly effective in treating mood disorders since the 1970s. I take it every day now, and when I take it I think of the melancholy reflection by the American poet Robert Lowell, who suffered from manic depressive psychosis in its most acute form until he started taking it:

> It's terrible to think that all I've suffered, and all the suffering I've caused, might have arisen from the lack of a little salt in my brain, and that if the effects of that salt had been known earlier, if I'd been given it earlier, I might have had a happy or at least a normal life, instead of this long nightmare.

I wouldn't say anything so radical, because even though I sometimes think it was, my life hasn't been one long nightmare. Still, I too belong to the group of bipolar patients who respond well to lithium. It makes my highs less high, my lows less low, and I'm so afraid to find myself once again in front of Raoul Dufy's little seascape that I'm ready to take it, obediently, for the rest of my life.

The terminal

I'm early, as usual: my flight for Lisbon is due to depart in an hour. As I've said, I have nothing against interstitial time, and I sit down to wait near my boarding gate in terminal 2 of Ponta Delgada Airport, on the Azores Islands. I've taken Cormac McCarthy's *Blood Meridian* out of my bag. I bought it for the trip because I'd mentioned McCarthy in my own book back when I was hospitalized at Sainte-Anne, more precisely when the young woman whom I didn't remember from the secure unit insisted that not only did we get to know each other there—very well, even—but also that we'd talked at length about Cormac McCarthy, of whom I was, like her, a passionate reader. So I thought it might be time to read him, you never know where a lead like that can take you. Maybe I'll stumble across something in this book that's absolutely essential to my own. That said, however talented Cormac McCarthy is, I have a hard time reading him. Having become, to my great surprise, almost exclusively a reader of poetry, I now find it very difficult to read novels. While reading the same page for the third time, which you could say went in one eye and out the other, I start to murmur a poem to myself as I often do—in this case one by Catherine Pozzi. I've already quoted a few of her verses, the ones I did my best to translate for Erica. Catherine Pozzi was a Parisian socialite between the wars, the wife of Édouard Bourdet—who was a famous playwright at the time—and the mistress of Paul Valéry, who made her very unhappy. Their affair inspired six loving, mystical poems that make her, in my opinion, an improbable and dazzling cross between the mystic philosopher Simone Weil and the Renaissance poet Louise Labé. And it's one of these poems, "Ave," that I recite to myself in the departure lounge:

> *O highest love, if I should die*
> *Without knowing how we came to be*
> *In what sun you dwelled*
> *In what past your time, in what hour*
> *   I loved you*

> *O highest love, that outlasts memory*
> *Fire without a hearth lighting my days*
> *In what fate you bound my tale*
> *In what sleep your glory was revealed*
> *   O my sojourn . . .*

I've got this far into the poem when I raise my head and see the Gemini woman, standing at the bar about ten yards away. I look at her without her seeing me, less moved than astonished. I came to the Azores for a conference but she lives in the Southern Hemisphere, and why she's here now is beyond me. We haven't seen or spoken to each other for three years. Thanks to the fact that my love fades when it's unrequited, I now rarely think about this woman whom I once passionately loved. She pays, and takes her coffee over to one of the white plastic stand-up tables arranged around the bar. That's when she sees me. I've had plenty of time to look at her without her seeing me, but not her. Or maybe she has, too. Maybe she saw me first, while I was trying to read Cormac McCarthy. In any case, our eyes meet without anything—absolutely anything—letting on that she's recognized me. Her gaze wanders over my row of chairs, absentmindedly taking in the people sitting here, then returns to her coffee cup. Since she's no longer looking at me I look at her, ready to adopt an expression of indifference if she looks up, and certain at the same time that she can feel me watching her. Her coffee finished, she leaves the stand-up table and heads over to a row of chairs quite far from mine. There aren't many passengers in the departure lounge, she can sit where she likes, and of course she's not going to take a seat next to me, but I wonder if she'll decide to sit facing me or if she'll face the other way. She sits a long way off but facing me, and like me she takes a book out of her bag and starts to read—without being able to concentrate any more than I can, at least so I imagine. What signal is she sending me by choosing—because it's obviously a choice—to face me instead of turning her back on me? Is this an invitation? What would happen if I got up, walked over to her, and took her by the hand? Would we walk out of the terminal together, the way we once walked out of the Gare de Genève-Cornavin, head over to one of the Sheraton or Sofitel hotels you can find at any airport, ask for a room at the front desk, go up together in one of the lifts, without a word, lock ourselves in that room of ours, and go under the radar for a few hours? I don't know. What I'm certain of, though, is that the scenario that's running through my head is also running through hers, and that she knows full well that it's also running through mine. And the knowledge that I have unlimited access to her thoughts and fantasies, and she to mine, makes the situation extraordinarily erotic. In fact, we don't even have to go to a hotel room: the way we looked at each other with feigned indifference during that half hour in the departure lounge, or didn't look at each other, the way each of us was alive to the other's presence without exchanging glances, the way we circled, feigned, dodged, and parried, was a way of making love whose power would have been weakened if we'd actually hit the sack. When we started boarding I let her go to the counter first, only getting up at the last minute, and I wondered what we'd do if chance sat us side by side, which—I was going to say fortunately—didn't happen. As I walked down the aisle toward the back of the cabin, I passed her. She was looking down at her book but I have no doubt that she felt me walk by, just inches away, and that like me she was stirred body and soul. During the flight I recited to myself the last stanzas of Catherine Pozzi's poem. I'd have liked some kind of telepathy to send these verses straight from my heart to hers:

When I shall be for myself lost
And divided to infinity
When I shall be infinitely ruptured
When the present that clads me
  betrays me

By the universe shattered in myriad fragments
From a thousand moments not yet assembled
From ashes to the heavens to nothing reduced
You shall remake for one strange year
  A single treasure

From a thousand bodies swept off by the day
You shall remake my name and my image
A lively unity, nameless and faceless
Heart of the spirit, center of the mirage
  O highest love.

The passengers exited the plane from the front, she got off well before I did. I thought that like me she'd have a connecting flight to Paris and that we'd continue the journey together, and I feared that this magical situation would become predictable, forced, tiresome. But either because Lisbon was her final destination or because she was going somewhere else, I didn't see the Gemini woman in the departure lounge for Paris, and haven't seen her to this day.

A quote

"For the moment, Patrice was there, cradling his dying wife, and however long she took, he would surely hold her until the end, until Juliette died safely in his arms. Nothing seemed more precious to me than that security, that certainty of being able to rest until the last moment in the embrace of someone who loves you completely. Hélène had told me what Juliette had said to their sister, Cécile, the previous day, when she could still speak. She'd said she was content: her quiet little life had been a success. At first I thought her words had been words of comfort; then I thought they were sincere, and in the end, true. I remembered Fitzgerald's famous dictum *All life is a process of breaking down*, and there I had to disagree. Or at least I didn't think it held true for every life. For Fitzgerald's, perhaps. For mine, perhaps—though I feared that more at the time than I do today. When Juliette passed judgment on her life, however, I believed her, and what led me to believe her is the image of that deathbed on which Patrice held her close. I told Hélène, You know, something happened. Only a few months ago, if I'd learned I had cancer and would soon die, if I'd asked myself the same question as Juliette—has my life been a success?—I could not have given the same answer. I'd have said no, I hadn't made a success of my life. I'd have said I'd succeeded in some things, had two handsome sons who were alive and well, and had written three or four books that gave form to what I was. I had done what I could, with my means and my shortcomings, and I'd fought to do so: that was something, after all. But the essential, which is love, would have escaped me. I was loved, yes, but I had not learned how to love—or hadn't been able to, which is the same thing. No one had been able to rest in complete confidence in my love and I would not rest, at the end, in anyone else's. That's what I'd have said at the news of my impending death, before the wave hit. And then, after the wave, I chose you, we chose each other, and now nothing's the same. You're here, close to me, and if I had to die tomorrow I could say like Juliette that my life has been a success."

"No one has been able to rest in my love, I will not rest in anyone else's"

Excuse me for quoting myself, and at such length. This last passage is from my book *Lives Other Than My Own*. I wrote it twelve years ago. Not only did I believe what I wrote there with all my heart, but I continued to believe it confidently for the next ten years, which were the best of my life. I knew that a love like that is rare, and that if you let it go by you'll be doomed to regret it and to the bitter taste of being too slow on the uptake. Where so many others failed, I thought I would succeed.

I didn't.

Gentle water

I continue not to die, as best I can. I continue not to die, but my heart is no longer in it. I believe I've used up my credit and nothing will happen anymore. And then one day something does happen. The unknown, which I both hope for and dread, takes on the form of a particular unknown woman, whom I start to get to know, and with whom I walk on a mountain path in Mallorca. The weather is nice, very mild for early spring. At a lodge where we've stopped to take a break and fill our water bottles, the woman in charge extols the virtues of this spring water that she calls *agua gentil*. In Spanish, *gentil* simply means fresh, or soft. The lodgekeeper is talking about the soft water, but for us that day "gentle water" becomes the code name for joy. A little later, we leave the path and rest on a large, flat white rock beside a stream. Very nearby, the young woman whom I'm starting to get to know and whom I'm already

starting to love tells me, the gentle water rises from the
earth. Back at home in the village, she does a bit of yoga.
Not the solemn, meditative type of yoga aimed at extin-
guishing the vritti, leaving samsara, or constructing a state
of wonder and serenity over a whole lifetime. No, not the
type of yoga to which I thought I'd dedicate this book,
solemnly explaining that it should not be confused with
vulgar gymnastics, but rather the type of yoga practiced
all over the world by young women who, like her, love it
precisely as a form of gymnastics, couldn't care less about
Patanjali, and have no desire whatsoever to leave samsara,
because samsara is also called life and, contrary to what
Patanjali and his followers think, life is good. Not *only*
good, of course, but good. And, considering all the things
that can be chalked up against me, I find life generous to
give me another chance. The young woman is now doing
a posture called *adhomukhavrikshasana*. She places her
hands flat on the ground near the wall and throws first
one leg and then the other up against the wall. She does
this without preparation, in a single movement, as if the
first thing she does when she sees a wall and she's in good
spirits—whoops!—is to throw her legs in the air, lightly,
carelessly, like a dance. Her summer dress falls around her
in a circle, revealing her tanned belly. Now she pulls her feet
away from the wall and points her toes skyward. Her feet are
up, her head is down, generally that doesn't put people in
a good light because the blood rushes to their head and
flushes their face, but not her, her upturned face is fresh
and joyful. Balancing on outstretched arms, her legs pointing to the sky, her belly in the air, she smiles at the man

she, too, is beginning to love, and this man, at this moment in her life and mine, is me, and I know that Raoul Dufy's little seascape is waiting for me, I know that I won't escape it, but on this day I don't care, on this day I'm completely happy to be alive.